Items should be returned on or before the last date
shown below. Items not already requested by other
borrowers may be renewed in person, in writing or by
telephone. To renew, please quote the number on the
barcode label. To renew online a PIN is required.
This can be requested at your local library.
Renew online @ **www.dublincitypubliclibraries.ie**
Fines charged for overdue items will include postage
incurred in recovery. Damage to or loss of items will
be charged to the borrower.

Leabharlanna Poiblí Chathair Bhaile Átha Cliath
Dublin City Public Libraries

Dublin City
Baile Átha Cliath

Brainse Mheal Ráthluirc
Charleville Mall Branch
Tel: 8749619

Date Due	Date Due	Date Due
04. JAN 12	24. 12	

My Dad Was Nearly James Bond

DES BISHOP

PENGUIN
IRELAND

PENGUIN IRELAND

Published by the Penguin Group
Penguin Ireland, 25 St Stephen's Green, Dublin 2, Ireland
(a division of Penguin Books Ltd)
Penguin Books Ltd, 80 Strand, London WC2R ORL, England
Penguin Group (USA) Inc., 375 Hudson Street, New York, New York 10014, USA
Penguin Group (Australia), 250 Camberwell Road, Camberwell, Victoria 3124, Australia
(a division of Pearson Australia Group Pty Ltd)
Penguin Group (Canada), 90 Eglinton Avenue East, Suite 700, Toronto, Ontario, Canada M4P 2Y3
(a division of Pearson Penguin Canada Inc.)
Penguin Books India Pvt Ltd, 11 Community Centre,
Panchsheel Park, New Delhi – 110 017, India
Penguin Group (NZ), 67 Apollo Drive, Rosedale, Auckland 0632, New Zealand
(a division of Pearson New Zealand Ltd)
Penguin Books (South Africa) (Pty) Ltd, 24 Sturdee Avenue,
Rosebank, Johannesburg 2196, South Africa

Penguin Books Ltd, Registered Offices: 80 Strand, London WC2R ORL, England

www.penguin.com

First published 2011

1

Set in 13.5/16 pt Garamond
Typeset by Palimpsest Book Production Limited, Falkirk, Stirlingshire
Printed in Great Britain by Clays Ltd, St Ives plc

A CIP catalogue record for this book is available from the British Library

ISBN: 978–1–844–88278–6

www.greenpenguin.co.uk

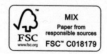

For my Mom, Michael John and Aidan
the show must go on.
And for Mr Paccione, do I get extra credit for this?

It was always a dream of mine to tell my dad's story. In the end I turned part of it into a one-man show called *My Dad Was Nearly James Bond*. The story was that my father had another life. He was an actor and a model in London, his friends had been famous people and, most exciting of all, he had once had an audition to play James Bond. But after I was born he gave all that up to give his children a more stable life than the unpredictable world of entertainment, and we settled in the semi-suburban world of my mother's home-town of Flushing, Queens, New York.

On 3 November 2009 my dad was diagnosed with stage four small cell lung cancer. I was inspired to tell his story then because I was so impressed by how he dealt with a terminal illness and what that did to our family.

When you do a show about cancer, everybody commends you for being able to deal with dark material in a light-hearted way. But the truth is that while my dad's illness was heart-breaking, it was not a time of darkness. For us, those last fifteen months were also a time of joy and laughter.

The real darkness lies in the part of my dad's past that I did not talk about in the show. It is the story of a boy whose mother was jailed after she tried to kill him, who was near destitute in his early twenties, and whose drinking could have destroyed him. That my dad survived all that and became a kind and hard-working father is even more remarkable than his encounters with fame during his years as a model and actor. And it puts his final struggle with cancer in an even more heroic light.

Some of his story I knew. Some more of it I found out during his illness. And the rest I'm still discovering. This is the real story of me and my dad, the man who was nearly James Bond.

PART ONE

Like Father . . .

It was Halloween 2009 and I could not have been having a nicer time with my nephew, my brother Michael John, my sister-in-law Maritza and my mother at Central Park Zoo. If anyone ever needed evidence of how oblivious I was of how much my life was about to change, I spent most of the day dressed as the Cat in the Hat from Dr Seuss. Although, as my father was such a performer, it was probably apt that the story should begin with me in costume.

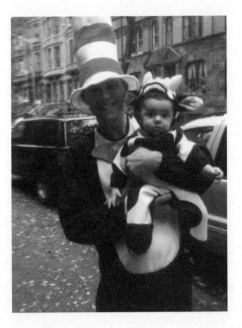

When my mother and I got back to the house, my father was still feeling terrible. He had had pneumonia for at least two weeks by that stage and he was not getting better. I felt bad for him because normally Halloween was a fun day for him and he always loved giving out candy to the trick-or-treaters throughout the early evening. I felt extra bad because I was really enjoying it. I loved all the surprised looks on the kids' faces as the Cat in the Hat answered the door. It was the first time I had been back in Flushing for Halloween since 1989 and I had forgotten how well New Yorkers celebrated the day.

I realized how sick my dad was when he did not want to have anything to do with the festivities. He was complaining about pains in his stomach and later that evening he started to experience shortness of breath. My mother had begun to entertain the idea of going to the hospital at around 4 p.m., but my dad was adamant that he did not want to go. Being an amateur doctor, I suggested he should eat some yoghurt as it might settle his stomach. In hindsight it is quite funny that all of us were trying to come up with simple cures to what turned out to be a terminal illness (I don't believe it has yet been proven that natural Greek yoghurt eases the symptoms of stage four lung cancer or metastases of the liver).

I went for a nap around half past six as I was tired from all the performing at the door. I passed out quickly as I was not really that worried at all about my dad. I was delighted with myself because I wasn't even home in order to see my sick dad; I had actually come home to spend time with my nephew. So I fell asleep, deeply content with the day we had just had.

I was woken by the strong New York accent of my cousin Jen, who is a nurse. I could hear her saying loudly, 'Awnt, you gotta get this guy to a hospital!' I could hear my dad protesting and then my mother coming up the stairs. I knew she was coming to wake me.

My mother is a chronic worrier who lives in a state of perpetual crisis, so I saw that familiar look of panic on her face, mixed with a hint of guilt that she had to disturb me from my sleep. Normally I might have been annoyed by my mother yet again taking a tiny drama and turning it into a crisis, but this time we had a genuine problem. Yoghurt had not done the trick and it was time to get real. I, along with my dad, had resisted going to the hospital until that point. I don't mind admitting that up till then I did not want the hassle. I had no idea how serious it was. But I could hear it in Jen's voice that she was genuinely worried.

Of course my mother said I did not have to come. I knew she meant 'I would love you to come'. So I packed my complaining dad into the car and off we went to what we know locally as Booth Memorial Hospital but which is now officially NY Hospital on Booth Memorial Avenue and Main Street in Flushing, Queens, NY.

No one wants to be in the emergency room of any hospital on Halloween night. If my father was writing this story, then I think there would be two chapters about that first night alone. There were people with horrible genuine injuries they sustained while drunk at Halloween parties, and people who had painted horrible fake injuries on their bodies coming in with asthma attacks and allergic reactions. You could not tell whether the injuries were real or applied! Most of them were way too loud for my dad, who felt terrible and did not sleep throughout the night. It is hard to get sleep when you feel like you want to die and the Grim Reaper is sitting next to you waiting to get his stomach pumped.

The next day my father was admitted. He had a small room with no windows, but it was totally private and he was very happy there after the trauma of the emergency room. He was asked a few alarming questions in those few days such as, 'Mr Bishop, are you a heavy drinker?' My dad took pride in telling them that he did not drink at all. By then, he had not had a drink for over thirty-five years.

For the next three days they sold us the story that he had very bad pneumonia and there was possibly something wrong with his liver. They say ignorance is bliss – and in my case it was true because, while we were sitting there watching the NY marathon on my dad's TV, I was not especially worried. I am almost embarrassed about that now, particularly because he was showing such glaring symptoms of lung cancer. I just did not know about them then.

I can't remember which of the initial three days it was, but we were told that he had a collapsed lung. I received the information with delight: I had a friend who had had a collapsed lung, so I knew that it was not a big deal. This must have been the Monday because he was scheduled for a bronchoscopy the following day, Tuesday, 3 November. Maritza, whose father had recently been diagnosed with pancreatic cancer, was the only one who sounded any real alarm. She had been looking things up online and knew that it was not a good symptom. I just put her concerns to the back of my mind. I was not even conscious that I was doing it.

The pulmonary specialist had requested a meeting with us after the bronchoscopy. At least three staff members of the hospital reminded us that it was important that we meet up with the specialist after my dad's test. My ignorance clearly turned to arrogance because I did not have a care in the world while I waited in the waiting room of the Lung Center. Ellen DeGeneres was on the TV and I struck up a conversation with an older man. I felt sorry for him as I could hear his shortness of breath.

My mother was with me. She was a wreck. She had obviously been on the internet and was expecting the worst. It was not until we were in the waiting room that she let me know that she was worried that this could be very bad. I told her that there was nothing to worry about. I was always telling my mother to chill out. Once again I thought she was panicking over nothing.

I know now that everyone was being overly nice to us. Even now I can see the reaction when I told the receptionist who we were and that the doctor had requested a meeting with us. We were VIPs on that day. When I think of all the doctors and nurses we dealt with in those few days, I wonder how they managed to pretend not to know what they knew. Now I know they knew and were just waiting for us to be told. They did an amazing job at keeping it from us. Those three days would have been hell if one of them had even planted the seed of worry in our minds. It was bad enough for my mother as it was.

The specialist tried to find a quiet place along a corridor. Normally he would have this chat in his office, he told us. His kind expression gave it away and, even before he said another word, I could feel my mother squeezing my arm more and more. The specialist was lovely. His main concern was finding more privacy for my mother. In the end there was nowhere else to go, and I just squeezed her close to me to protect her from the public as they strolled past.

'Malignancy' was the word he used. My mother squeezed my arm so hard it actually hurt me and then the pressure eased as she moved her hand to her mouth and started sobbing. I could feel the tears welling deep inside me too, but I tried to keep them down long enough to hear what the specialist was saying.

I asked if that was why they had been asking about his liver, and he said he could not say for certain but it was most likely metastases. The rest is not important, other than that I am pretty sure he told us that the prognosis was not good. I think he used the word 'terminal', but I can't be sure. I know that I did not leave the conversation with any hope. I thanked him.

I don't even know why, but I had an immense desire to be outside. My mother was crying in a way I had never heard before. I was literally holding her up. I wanted to cry too, but I was not going to do it inside that hospital. I pleaded with my mother to just try to walk. She was close to being physically unable to move.

It was quite a way to go to get out of the Lung Center. We had gone only some of the way when my mother saw a chair outside the cafeteria we had sat in many times over the last few days. It had been a great place to take a break from the room and the coffee there was surprisingly good. She begged me to let her sit down. As we sat there she was crying and I could see everyone looking at us as they went inside for their lunch. The normality of their lives seemed an affront. We are not safe here, I thought to myself.

I dragged her up. I told her that I was going to get her out of that hospital whether she liked it or not. In my mind, not making it outside meant defeat. I begged her to keep walking. I wanted to get outside and to be able to open the floodgates where no one else was around. I could feel all her weight in my arms as we finally made it to the door. It was a beautiful day and there were only a few clouds in the sky. I scanned the scene and saw, down a grassy slope, a bench facing the wall of the hospital. The bench was well below street level and it faced away from the street, so even if people could see us we could pretend they weren't there.

My mother said to me that we were not supposed to walk on the grass. I didn't give a shit about the grass. All that mattered was getting to a safe place. The safety was an illusion, but the desire for it was intense.

We cried together on that bench for a long time. My mother's repeated cry was, 'What are we going to do?' I told her that, no matter what happened, I would look after her forever.

I could not believe that we were having this conversation. I had thought many times about what would happen if one of my parents got sick, but I did not see it coming this fast. Now I was squeezing my mother, trying to protect her from the world. I cried more for my mother than anything else. Her world had just fallen apart and all I could do was hold her. Sad as I was, I had never felt closer to my mother. Later that day I took a picture of the bench on my phone because I wanted to remember that moment always.

She told me on the bench that she could not handle this and that I was going to have to deal with it. For the time being she abdicated her role as a parent. I was now the parent of my parents. In fact, I had felt that transition almost immediately after I had heard the news and when I was carrying my mother out of the hospital.

While we were still on the bench, I left a message on Michael John's phone and I left it a while to call my other brother Aidan because he would have been alarmed by how early it was, back in Ireland. I called my cousin Kevin to get the word out to the family. It just helped a little to try immediately to organize things or at least get into the drama of it for a minute after crying for a spell. We then decided that it was time to go see my dad.

I didn't actually cry again until I saw my brother Michael John. I left my dad to meet him on the street to give him the pass to the hospital room about an hour later. The minute we saw each other we broke down. It's strange the way certain things just set you off, but in this case I guess it's easy to see why. We were both thinking: Dad is dying.

*

I was told by the pulmonary guy that I would be the one to tell my dad the news, so I was trying to prepare myself. The minute I saw him I knew there was no need, as it was clear that he had been told. He looked so defeated, sitting on the edge of the bed. He half turned his head to us when we arrived and then looked back down through his exposed knees to the tip of his toes just touching the floor. It looked as if he had shrunk because the height of the hospital bed did not allow his feet to touch the ground. There he sat like a child, with his legs, all swollen from water retention, dangling, most likely feeling that his time was up.

He told us that his heart specialist had been in to see him. My father had a great relationship with his heart doctor and I guess he had asked the pulmonary guy to let him know the results straight away.

'He said that they found something, so I asked him to tell me if it was bad. He said it does not look good, so I asked him, was it the big C, and he said it looks like it. Not good, man. Not good.'

My father always repeated things for emphasis. This was a big one. His close friend Ed Higgins had died from lung cancer only a couple of years before. Ed had had a horrific time and fought until the very end with no real quality of life. Since then my dad would always say, 'If I ever get the big C, they won't do to me what they did to Ed Higgins.' He always used to say to me after he came back from the doctor over the last ten years, 'I told him I don't care what it is once it's not the big C.' So to my dad this really was 'not good, man'.

I think he said he might have asked the doctor about some of his options. He said a few more things and then went silent. There was nothing left to say.

I was glad a doctor had already told him, because on the

long walk back to his room I had been dreading telling him the news. I sat down next to him on the bed and put my arm around him and, unexpectedly, he just dropped his head on to my chest. He did not cry but he just rested his head there for ages. I held him and stroked his coarse, grey hair. I said nothing but I just tried to scream silently from every pore in my body, 'Everything is going to be all right.' I was not yet a parent, but at that moment I felt like my father's father – trying to protect him from the terror life had just thrown at him. It was the most intimate moment I had ever had with him. No words were exchanged.

I wrote this when I got home that evening:

> From the cradled to the cradler,
> I held his head in my chest
> And I wished that he would fight
> For my sake.

Defeat and surrender are closely related, and I felt defeat in my father that day. I surrendered immediately to the reality that my father was going to die. I pondered only death as an outcome. To me it was imminent.

But my mother was not prepared to give up at all. She could hardly remember a life without my father and she was not ready to even consider a future without him. The spirit to fight came first from her and soon after from him. He was only defeated that first day because he was tired. Despite appearing to accept that he was shortly going to die, he would soon realize he was not yet ready to go. Neither of them was ready to give up.

2

My father always wanted to keep everybody happy because what everybody else thought of him was paramount. Even how he ended up raising his family in New York begins with him trying to please someone. After my parents married in New York in 1973 they returned to London, where my father had had a successful modelling career before moving to New York in 1969. In early 1975 my mother's father, whom we later knew as Pop Pop, died. Soon after, my grandmother moved to London to be with my mom during her pregnancy (with me). My father loved my grandmother so much. For

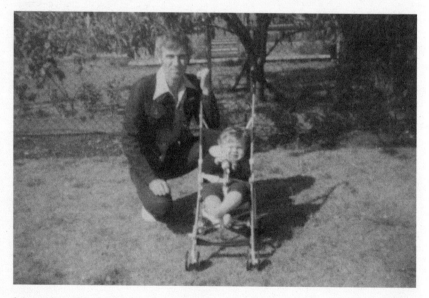

him she was the perfect woman – she was from West Cork, loved to drink and loved all my dad's stories – and he would have done anything for her. She spent most of her time trying to get them to move back to New York. My mother was happy to stay in London for a while longer, but my nan worked on my dad. In the end he wanted to keep her happy and, though life was good on the King's Road in Chelsea, I was brought back to Queens at three weeks of age, having been registered by my mother as an American Born Abroad with the US Embassy in London.

We lived with Nanny until 1978. By then, both she and my father were members of Alcoholics Anonymous and they had very similar circles of friends. He was starting a new life and was getting to know the network of sober Irish in Queens, and these would be the people I would know as his best friends all my life.

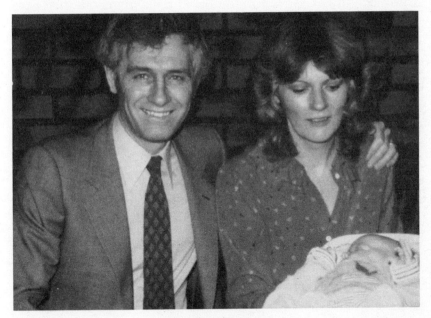

Aidan's christening

My brother Michael John was born during the blizzard of 1978. By that time my parents were looking for a place to live, and by the end of 1978 we had moved into the house that became our home on 47th Avenue and 188th Street in the Auburndale section of Flushing. Aidan came along in February 1980.

My earliest memories of the house are of horrible green carpets and awful yellow paint. My father spent the next few years stripping paint from any bit of wood he could find. It was tough stripping away the bad taste of the 1970s, but by the time I was seven the house was all stained wood and white paint. My father would paint the walls of the world white if he could.

I was not the child of a model or an actor, I was the son of a retail man. I now realize that as he entered his forties and settled into family life, my father faced the fear that ageing can bring to people who look good for a living. He had one child and the desire for more, and he knew that his work was not stable enough for the life he wanted to provide. The recession had kicked in and it was a hard time to find work, but he had connections in Barneys, the high-end Manhattan clothing store, because he had modelled their clothes many times. The manager in Barneys told him that the only position he had was folding garments and, without telling my mother, he took the job. He never admitted to her that he was starting in such a lowly position.

He didn't have to hide his inferior position for long and he quickly ended up a department manager in Barneys. He was still in Barneys when my parents bought our house on 188th Street. It was in Barneys also that he met a headhunter who would become a great friend of my parents and the man responsible for my dad's retail career progressing. He encouraged my dad to keep going for bigger and better jobs, but after my dad eventually became general manager of another high-end Manhattan store, Burberrys, my mother made him promise that he would not change jobs again. All this change unsettled her, as my dad's educational history was very skimpy, and as he progressed in retail he had pretended to have a better education than he actually had. They were both paranoid about this coming back to bite him if he pushed it too far.

I assume he got caught up in the business of building a new career and was initially quite satisfied that he had progressed so quickly from such a lowly position. Later on in life he would see what he had achieved as not very impressive and would focus more on the life he left behind rather than the life he had created for his family.

My earliest memories of my dad working are from his time in Abraham & Straus, a large department store out on Hempstead Turnpike in Nassau County, Long Island. He had a low-level management position there after being headhunted from Barneys. My dad hated it out there. It was a step too far from the city life he had known for so long. It was tough enough being a nine-to-five dude; being out in Long Island just made it worse. But he had been offered a manager's job, so he took it as a stepping stone.

Hempstead Turnpike was an eight-lane road, a classic suburban American boulevard created for a world where the car was king. Crossing it at a set of traffic lights was taking your life in your hands: pedestrians were intruders in the commuter world of Long Island. All along it was a world of small shopping malls with massive car parks. My dad did not have a driving licence and never drove, so we often went out to pick him up. We had a Plymouth Duster which was orange, so everyone thought it was the car from *The Dukes of Hazzard*.

If my mother was not picking him up he had a tough journey home, as public transport was not great around there. It was probably a quarter-mile walk from A&S to the turnpike through a desolate car park. I can only imagine the thoughts he must have had out there in a world of cars during the long, hot, humid New York summers – the only one walking, the only one waiting for the bus, the only one who could not drive. He was a city man lost in the deep suburbs. He did not belong there among the franchise steakhouses and the Burger Kings. He was a stand-up guy lost in a drive-through world.

He loved getting back to his boys though. When he came home we would beg him to play 'Batman'. I don't know why we called it Batman. I think Batman was on Saturday morning cartoons back then and we were big fans. The game had nothing to do with Batman, though. All we did was run at my dad, who was sitting on his bed, and he would flip us over,

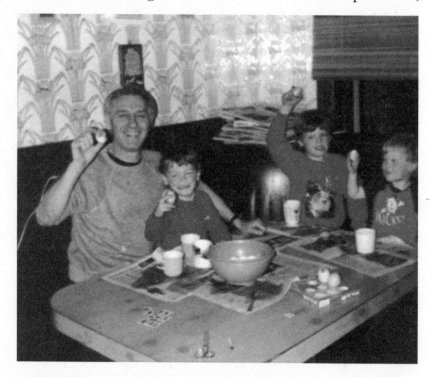

his head. Sometimes he could not do it because throughout his life he struggled with back pain caused by an accident when he was a young man. The more he threw us, the more we loved it. He may have regretted it because my parents' bed would become our playground for the rest of our young lives. First it was the bat cave, later it was a trampoline, and eventually it became a World Wrestling Federation ring. Even worse for my parents' bed: their dresser became the top rope and often we would jump high off it on to the bed, impersonating Jimmy Superfly Snuka and Ricky the Dragon Steamboat. I don't think there was a day when one of us did not leave that room crying.

We were his three boys. To Americans that's kind of funny because there was a huge series in the 1960s called *My Three Sons*. We were happy to be those sons and we loved our dad being around. He would call me Dessie Doodle, Michael John was Mikey John and Aidan was Aidee Aid Aid. We were his three 'scallywags'. We never knew what a scallywag was and neither did anyone else in the neighbourhood, but it was such a great word. It was the first thing many guys said to us when they came to my dad's wake: 'He always called me a scallywag. What the hell is it?'

3

When you are a kid you always think your dad is the coolest dad in the world. It turns out that we were not the only ones. At my dad's wake I asked anyone who wanted to say a few words to come up. A friend of mine, Joe Lane, said he was always aware that Mr Bishop was different from the other dads because he was good-looking and always seemed interested in you. Even the kids in the area felt my father's charm. My dad had that effect on everyone. He made everyone feel great.

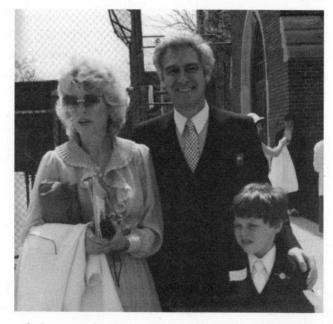

Most of the people I knew in St Kevin's parish were white Catholics: mostly Italian and Irish Americans and some Greek Orthodox kids who had moved out from Astoria, Queens. There were other races too, but those three predominated. I would call it a working-class area now, but back then we were told that we were middle class. Americans don't like the term 'working class'; they might say 'blue-collar' instead. I think it would be fair to say our neighbourhood was bleached blue-collar, as many tradesmen in unions in New York did very well and had high standards of living while keeping a working-class sensibility. There were a lot of cops and firemen in our area too. There were also a lot of immigrants that we called 'off the boat'. They spoke Italian and Greek in the house and the kids were bilingual. Off the boat was an important matter in our area because we all thought we were Irish or Italian or Greek. But really we were hyphens: Irish-Americans, Greek-Americans, Italian-Americans. But some people's parents had no hyphens because they were off the boat. The genuine article.

The Giourakis family would speak only Greek. You could hear their mother shouting from across the garage rooftops, *'NIKO! GIANNI! ELEA THO!'* It means 'Come here' or 'Come home'. We heard it every day. Angelo Messina's mother struggles with English to this day. Every time I meet her I think she could have been off the boat yesterday. She always seemed to be cooking or hanging out laundry. *'ANGELO, MANGI, MANGI!'* My friend P.J.'s mother had a bell and would ring it when it was time for his dinner – *'COOOOOMMMMMEE AND GET IT!'* – and he would run home like a cattle hand. His grandmother came over sometimes and I could not understand her when she was speaking Italian. My grandmother would come over and he could not understand her when she was speaking English because she never lost her West Cork accent. My nan spoke so fast it was like she was auctioning cattle. I don't think she understood herself sometimes. The neighbourhood was so diverse and family orientated, it would had made the Statue of Liberty cry with pride.

Our street was a row of mock-Tudor terraced houses without any back gardens. Instead there were communal driveways at the back which gave everyone access to their garages. We referred to them as 'the alley' even though we were talking about a few of them. The neighbourhood was criss-crossed by these alleyways, many of which could be accessed without crossing any streets. This was perfect for us kids because it created places to play with no traffic. Crossing the street was forbidden without permission for quite a long time, so I played in the three alleys that were accessible. These alleyways became a baseball field in the summer and a football field in the winter. Eventually my best friend and neighbour, Shannon Docherty, got a basketball hoop put up over her garage, and basketball also became a big game.

We hid in the gaps between garages, made forts from the underside of porches where the garbage cans were stored; we climbed the roofs to get balls, we danced in the puddles left by the torrential summer thunderstorms even though our parents told us we would get polio. We turned stoops into ball games with new rules every day; we umpired our whiffle-ball games, refereed our two-hand touch football games and argued over every call. 'You only got me with one hand, that's bullshit.' We drove Mr Benari crazy. He was the grumpy old man on the corner of 189th. He complained every day about the noise we made and even called the cops on us one time for playing in the street. But if you want to live around quiet kids, then don't buy a house in Queens. We said he should live in a garbage can and we called him Oscar the Grouch.

And we fought all the time. P. J. Puma was my other best friend, and any time we were together we were either playing or fighting. He was a year older than me so he always won the fights. Within ten minutes we would be friends again and I would continue to play with streaks down my dusty face where my tears had left their mark. I did not have to worry about ever actually winning a fight against P. J. because his sister was always beating him up because she was older. In the alley somebody older was always beating up someone younger. The beatings got passed down, like a hot potato of violence, but when I look back I can't recall a single ounce of pain. We were all made of rubber.

We didn't worry about the sun, hydration, who hit who, falling, kidnapping or even germs. We would have eaten cookies we found on the ground if you kissed it up to God. We played outside all the time. Our parents never worried about where we were. When it was time for dinner they would shout or send some other kid to tell you that your mom said dinner was ready. A parent's presence at the top of the alley was always ominous; it was the only thing we worried about. Mine would turn up a lot. I was often in trouble as I was a pretty hyper kid.

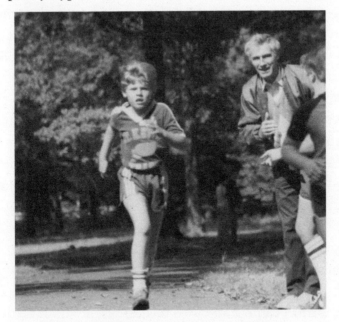

My dad urging me on from the sidelines.

We were all pretty hyper kids. Our generation of youngsters had a lot of freedom back then. There must have been thirty of us in our immediate area and we filled the place with energy, laughter and tears from sun-up to sun-down when we were not at school. When we got too old to play, the streets became much quieter because we were hiding – either getting drunk or making out.

You could see the contrast between my dad and other dads really clearly on the sidelines of our soccer games on 73rd Avenue. There in a line of dads – lots of fat fathers in tracksuits and their wife-beater T-shirts – and then my dad in a tweed cap with an umbrella by his side. The Queens dads would shout, 'Go get him, Carlos. Come on, offense!' My dad would shout, 'Watch your house, support him, unload it, get into space.' The other coaches would say, 'Just go out there and do your best.' My father would say, 'It's a passing game, when not in possession get in position.' He would often get into the car majorly annoyed by his perception of the American dad's ignorance of football. 'Hey, Michael John, what are they on about – "Double team him!" It's not bloody basketball.'

Although I was an average soccer player, my father suddenly decided, a few years after I had started playing, that I had a talent for goalkeeping. I think I was around seven or eight at the time. I can't remember what I actually did, but I recall how everyone went on about how during a particular game I had saved a one-on-one breakaway. My dad was delighted and I was thrilled to have impressed him. Suddenly I was a star goalkeeper.

My high standing did not last very long. Soon after that I faced a team that included one of my Italian classmates, Giancarlo Petrucelli. Giancarlo was the best player in our age group. Not only that, but he was really big. He had probably hit puberty by the age of seven – those Italians get hairy very early. Anyway, I was definitely afraid that day. I did not want to play in goal against Giancarlo, plain and simple. I must have moaned a lot, but in the end my father forced me to go in the goal.

Nothing could stop Giancarlo. I think he scored two goals within the first five minutes. I said I felt sick and walked off. I can't remember exactly what my father said, but it was something along the lines of calling me a baby in front of everyone who was there. My father very rarely blew his cool in front of other people – it was just not his way – so for him to show his anger publicly meant he was really pissed off. I was very embarrassed, but so was he. He did not want all the people who were watching the game seeing one of his boys being weak. With my dad it was all about the people who were watching.

I wandered off towards the woods that bordered the soccer fields while the match continued. There was an abandoned tunnel under the Clearview Expressway near the soccer fields at Cunningham Park where we were playing. When I was a boy you had to go through the woods to get to it. It was full of garbage, covered in graffiti and quite scary to a boy. Though I didn't know it then, this was the Vanderbilt Highway, a toll road created by the Vanderbilts to get the rich folk from their Long Island mansions back into New York City. It was made famous as the road that they use in *The Great Gatsby* to travel between the city and East Egg.

I can still see myself walking to that place through those woods on the edge of the wilderness. I had no perception then that, a few streets away, there was an end to them. I thought I could get lost in them and never come out. I walk over the brown leaves that covered the path. I can hear them crackling under me, crispy and dead in the dry November cold. I can see my breath on the dark silver light. I can see myself sitting in the dark tunnel and listening to the echo of my voice and trying to make different noises. It is really scary here. It is really lonely but I don't want to leave.

The tunnel was a place to hide out after the disappointment of letting my father down. I felt real bad about that, but I also thought he was an asshole. I hated him at that moment. It was the first time I became aware of not liking my dad. Worse, though, I was so disappointed in myself. He was worried about what everybody else thought, but I was only worried about what he thought.

My dad's disgust and disappointment that day had a profound effect on me. I never really played soccer after that. I definitely did not go back into goal ever. I would later realize that my dad was keen that we perform well in sports. He had been a sports star, so he expected the same from us. To the end of his life my dad would say that I could have been a brilliant 'keeper. There were too many 'could haves' and 'should haves' in my dad's life.

4

My father began to speak openly about death very soon after his diagnosis. I think he thought he was dying during those first few days. He said that he wished a few times he would die because he was feeling so terrible. He began chemo almost straight away in the hospital, and though he had some side effects his condition began to improve.

There must be something instinctual about accepting death, because he seemed to accept it more in his first few weeks of being sick than he did a year later, after much chemotherapy. In fact, in the end he refused to accept that he had no chance of beating the cancer. Thank God he didn't give in to his first impulse to accept death, because we would never have had the extraordinary time we spent together.

There is so much I could write about the amazing times I shared with my dad right after he got sick. Our family became extremely close around that period. There was an incredible love between all of us and I really enjoyed it, despite the illness and the sadness. I felt a terrible pity for my dad, at times seeing him uncomfortable in the hospital; but more than that I doted over him. He looked almost cute in his hospital bed and there was a baby-like sense about him; I just wanted to hug him and stare at him all the time.

I used to love washing him in the hospital. There were so many lovely things about it. His gratitude was so flattering and so endearing. It was obvious that he felt much better after a good bed wash. It was a nice feeling for me to feel useful and be able to look after my family in this way. He would look over at my mother and say, 'Isn't this lovely, Eileen.' Or look up at me and say, 'I am so lucky to have sons like you.'

Within two weeks of my dad's diagnosis it was my thirty-fourth birthday and I spent my birthday in the hospital room, looking after my dad. So many of my friends have kids now, and I don't, so this was the first time I was responsible for looking after someone in this way. There was a tenderness in being this close to my father; there was no awkwardness between us, and there was no awkwardness within the family. We showered my father with love, and it was the most remarkable atmosphere.

I felt so necessary, filling up his wash bowl and rubbing him down with the cloth. There was something about wash-ing under his armpits that made me feel so good: I guess because I thought it was making him feel clean. It was almost as if I was trying to wash away the horror of the first few days and make him feel like he was back in the game. I would give him gentle massages and put a hot cloth on his skin. I was trying to copy some of the tricks I had picked up from too many days killing time in hotel spas while I was on tour. It might be one of the only positive legacies of the Celtic Tiger. I was trying to pamper him as much as I could.

I will never forget the sound of my father's unkempt stubble. I felt I could hear each individual hair as it was released from the backs of my fingers as I stroked his face. I can still smell the moisturizer we used to rub on his legs to stop the skin from cracking. The best of all, though, was the way he used to feel so much better after it and was very vocal in his praise and gratitude. Despite the fact that I was now parenting my parent, I still had the delight of a son who is impressing his dad. It was lovely.

I learned many things about my dad's taste in music during

his stay in the hospital. To pass the time I used to show my dad videos on my iPhone of stuff he was into when he was younger. For my dad, the fact that he could watch videos from a device in my hand blew his mind. He really got into it. He was a huge Moody Blues fan, a fact which I had never known before. He sang along to 'Nights in White Satin' in his hospital bed. We watched John Lennon and 'The Peanut Vendor' by Stan Kenton, which I had never heard of, but my dad remembered going to see him in London. We also listened to 'Morning Has Broken': Dad told me that he had thought of this song on his first morning in his new hospital room. From the window, there was a distant view of the Manhattan skyline. Dad had been up all night, and as he watched the morning come to life he sang that song to himself. I know that at that time he was already thinking about death. (When my dad died, my brother told me that he knew he was going to die in the morning because of the way he talked about singing 'Morning Has Broken' a year and a half before.)

Singing was a big thing for my dad. He loved to sing. Whenever he talked about his mother he would say the same thing: 'She loved to sing.' When I think of it, that is all he ever said about her when we were young. Even my cousins in Midleton would say that about her: 'She had a great singing voice.' When my father told me he went to see her before she died, he said that they just sat down and sang the old songs from Cork.

5

When we were young it was hard to pin down exactly who my dad was. He was born in 1936 of an English father and an Irish mother – so, I often joke, he was born to hate himself. His Irish identity was a huge part of him, even though he sounded and acted more like an English gent. His mother, Hannah Ryan, was from Midleton, County Cork, and she had moved to England with her sister Peggy. My paternal grandfather, Stanley Bishop, was from Sussex.

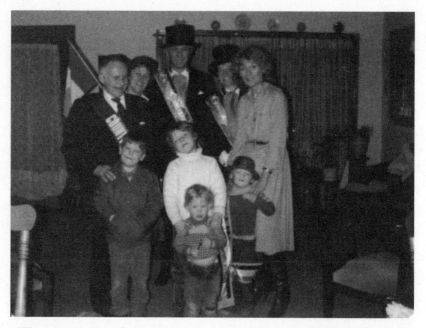

We were so into being Irish. I mean, look at us: it was not even St Patrick's Day, we were just going to Mass!

Growing up, I thought I was the son, grandson and great-grandson of men who fought in the British Army. This is despite that fact we were brought up to believe that we were Irish first and foremost. My mother was strongly Irish-American. O'Hare was her maiden name. Her father was from County Down, and she was quite republican too. She worked for O'Dwyer & Bernstein, a law firm that often represented republican prisoners on the run from Britain. As kids we marched for County Down in the St Patrick's Day Parade, and we got goosebumps when we would see the 'Get the Brits Out of Ireland' banners hanging from office blocks all along 5th Avenue.

My dad liked to write Irish songs and, sometime in the 1980s, he was even awarded the No. 1 song of the year on Fordham Radio, the Irish station in New York, with a song about children in Northern Ireland called 'Run Children, Run'. I am not sure if it made any money, but all the profits went to Project Children Northern Ireland.

Then again, in his job in Burberrys, he was incredibly British. He would talk about soccer with some of the other English guys and he would be like a different person. He would always tell the same story that the Arsenal footballer Bob McNab said to him, 'that in his day Georgie Best was unplayable'. I must have heard that story a thousand times. He would become almost cockney when he was on a roll with these guys. At work, it was better to be English. We could always tell who he was talking to on the phone at home because he used a different accent, depending on where the person was from. My dad was always who he thought you wanted him to be.

It was also hard to know much about my dad's past because his mother lived in England, in a nursing home, and his sister Joan did too until she moved to Australia to follow her children when they emigrated there. All my relatives were on my mother's side and we were all very close. My mother's mother had seventeen grandchildren, and when we were young we saw each other every holiday. All my cousins loved my dad and they never really saw him as their uncle through marriage, so it was easy to just feel like this was our entire family. I had no connection to my dad's family and his past, so the scant information I had seemed to be enough.

When he was eighteen my father joined the British Army. I don't know much about the details, but I know he was in the Army Physical Training Corps. I did not know much about that either; but a few years ago I met Northern Irish comedian Roy Walker, whom I recognized from *Catchphrase*, and he said he had also been in the Army Physical Training Corps and he seemed very proud to have been a part of that. I know that my dad served in Malaysia, and I believe there were a few decent fights in that one. He was not much for talking about his time in the army, as I think he was paranoid about what his Irish friends might think about it. It was an important period of his life, however, in which he received the only real education he ever had. Boxing and gymnastics were a big part of his life in the army and he also played football for the Sussex Regiment.

When he finished with the army, fitness continued to be central to his life, and he even tried to make a living doing gymnastic exhibitions. I know he also had a window-cleaning business, and I think for a time he was happily living in Bexhill-on-Sea in East Sussex, his home town. Then one day while training on a trampoline he landed the wrong way and was propelled into the air at an angle. He landed flat on his back on the bar of the trampoline and broke his back. I heard him tell the story many times. Sometimes he said he had been drinking; I can't say for certain. He ended up having three spinal fusions and was in the hospital for the best part of a year. It was the end of his career as a gymnast.

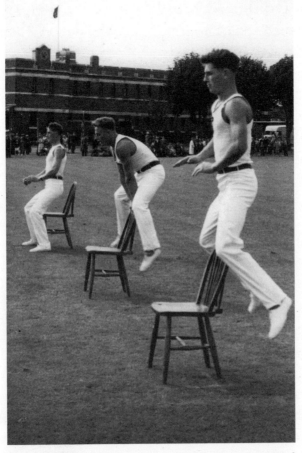

My father is the one at the front of the picture. My dad was more than just handsome, he was seriously fit.

Dad always said that at some stage during his recovery a friend of his who had moved to London suggested he should move to London too and become a model. It was easy to see why he would have suggested this, as my dad was definitely model material. When he was well enough he moved up there and eventually ended up with the model agency, Scotty's. Their client list in the late 1960s was pretty impressive and included George Lazenby. The industry was really just getting off the ground then, so it was an exciting time to be part of it.

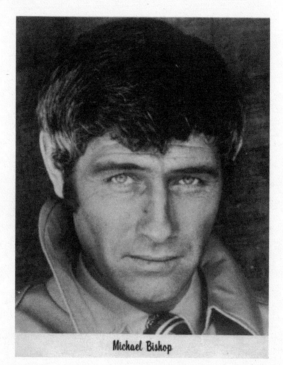

Michael Bishop

I always think this picture says it all. He was an incredibly good-looking man in his day. Don't get me wrong, I am happy with my own looks, but I can't help looking at this picture sometimes and thinking, 'You kept a couple of genes in your pocket there, you greedy bastard!'

He was a very successful model, and various relations over the years have told me stories about how they would be waiting in the Underground in the 1960s and all of a sudden they would realize that their cousin was staring at them from every poster. I think he really wanted to be an actor, though, and I would imagine he must have thought he had a chance, seeing how successful he was as a model. He had bit parts in *The Day of the Triffids* and *Zulu* and was in a film called *Last of the Long-haired Boys* that I don't think was ever released. He did some adverts too, but I only know of ones that came after he had met my mother.

Then came the story that we would be told over and over again. It turns out that Scotty's provided a lot of the men who auditioned for the part of James Bond in *On Her Majesty's Secret Service*. I think it must have been a tough job finding a replacement for Sean Connery; Roger Moore could not do it as he was committed to *The Saint*, and Timothy Dalton had decided he was too young. The casting director had decided he wanted to cast a model. Mike Bishop was one of those who read for the part. The only fact I know for certain is that Scotty's was definitely a part of the casting story. According to research I've done, my dad was not one of the main contenders – but that is not the way he told the story when we were kids. In fairness to him, it was really my cousin Ira (the husband of my mother's first cousin Maureen) who let the story grow. He sold televisions for a living in Greenwich Village and was obsessed with film. He loved the story and would bring it up every Christmas, Thanksgiving and Easter. He always said that Lazenby beat him to it, so in my mind my dad and Lazenby had been sitting outside an office, waiting to be told the news; it was that close.

Perhaps there are some Bond fans who are thinking that my dad was lucky, as it is commonly held that George Lazenby was the worst James Bond. My dad never saw it as lucky: if George Lazenby was the worst James Bond, then he was worse than the worst James Bond.

Bond fans need to be told now that there are no James Bond jokes or stories in this book. I have never actually watched an entire James Bond film because we were not allowed to watch James Bond in our house. My dad hated James Bond and would always make us change the channel if a Bond movie came on. I don't think he wanted to be reminded of what might have been in the late 1960s.

The other reason why the legend of his near-miss grew was because my dad was in a production of John B. Keane's *Sive* in London when the hunt for the new Bond was on. He sometimes said that the Bond people had seen him in the play and that is how he got the audition.

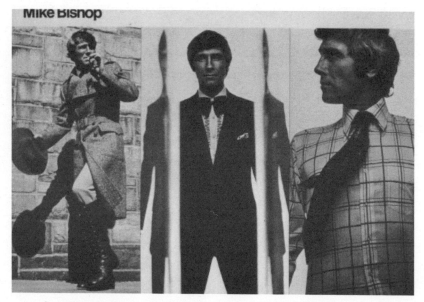

Mike Bishop

Any man who can pull off wearing boots like that could definitely have been considered for James Bond.

My cousins in Midleton always said they had seen a newspaper article about him being up for the Bond role and that a woman had the article in a pub somewhere in town, though

I've never seen it. Either way, the Midleton cousins held on to that story. To them, their nephew and cousin was nearly James Bond. They must have told everybody because, a few years later when my dad visited Midleton, the local paper ran a story, which I have seen, headlined 'BBC Star Visits Midleton', accompanied by a picture of my dad.

I was always very critical of the embellished stories my dad told, but really he was just playing to the crowd. The family wanted the stories just as much as he did.

It seemed as if everything was going great for my dad in London as the 1960s were coming to a close. He was part of the fashionable and arty '60s London scene of actors, models, artists and hangers-on. With his girlfriend Valerie he set up a beauty salon in Chelsea and the opening was quite a society event. In today's world he would have been turning up in the social columns and the pages of *OK!* and *Hello!* magazine. He and Valerie hung out with a heavy-drinking crowd. His close friends were actors Dudley Sutton, Donal McCann and Dermot Harris, the brother of Richard Harris. Years later Dermot died from alcoholism. (Dad was also friends with Dermot's wife Cassandra who, coinciden-tally, would end up playing Countess Lisl von Schlaf in *For Your Eyes Only* and who married Pierce Brosnan, who later became James Bond.)

Back when I was a teenager I always doubted my father's name-dropping of people he knew from his drinking days in London. The best stories he told in later years were the tales of his drinking escapades with the painter Francis Bacon. I did not believe them at first. My dad could do an impression of him, which meant nothing to me when I was young, but when I watched a documentary about Bacon in recent years it turned out his mimicry was spot on.

I first got an inkling that maybe my dad wasn't all talk on my eighteenth birthday in November 1993. I was in Blackrock College repeating my Leaving Cert. and the dean, Fr Reilly, came to tell me that I had special permission to listen to *Late Date* on RTÉ Radio One, as there would be a request played for me by the DJ, Val Joyce. The request was from Donal McCann, who wanted to wish the oldest son of his good friend Mike Bishop a happy eighteenth. (Val Joyce played a Tom Petty track as he said it was the only thing he had that would suit a boy of my age.) It just so happened that Donal McCann was on the cover of the edition of *Juno and the Paycock* I was studying for the Leaving Cert. The penny only dropped two weeks later when I saw his name credited as the man in the picture: my dad's buddy was on the cover of my textbook, so he must be famous.

My dad's career had a lot of momentum in London, so I am not sure why he decided to leave it all and go to New York in 1969. It seemed a glamorous life but somehow he had become disillusioned with it, and when Gerry Ford of the Ford Modelling Agency came to take some of London's models back to New York, my father jumped at the chance. Like many people in the entertainment world from Britain the lure of cracking America was too strong. My dad would later regret that decision because all the work he had done in London to build his reputation was wasted. He never really had any acting success in New York, and they would quickly forget him in London.

Though we were not children of the entertainment industry, I guess if there was one unique thing about being the children of a man who once modelled for the Ford Modelling Agency it was that . . .

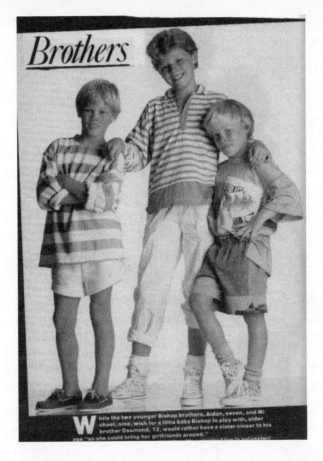

Brothers

While the two younger Bishop brothers, Aidan, seven, and Michael, nine, wish for a little baby Bishop to play with, older brother Desmond, 12, would rather have a sister closer to his age "so she could bring her girlfriends around."

. . . we modelled for the Ford Modelling Agency. From the age of eight to twelve I used to work as a child model, as did my brothers. There is not much to say about it, but I always like this photo because it was actually about us. We were not just some generic kids in a catalogue. This was a feature in *Children's Business* about 'Brothers in the Modelling Game'. They even asked us a few questions. It says underneath, 'While the two younger Bishop brothers, Aidan, seven, and Michael, nine, wish for a little baby Bishop to play with, older brother Desmond, twelve, would rather have a sister closer to his age so she could bring her girlfriends around.'

Desperate to be funny already at twelve.

6

Most of our summers were spent out at the Mineola Pool Club in Long Island. In Nassau County many of the towns had a pool club for local residents. Some of the towns near Queens also allowed non-residents to join for an increased fee. This meant that many families from our area drove out on the Long Island Expressway on hot summer days to spend the day there. We had chosen Mineola because some people my mother grew up with, the Lennons, also went out there.

Nanny used to come out with us to the pool club most days, which was kind of a nightmare because both my parents smoked, as did Nanny. So we would all pile into the 1980 Ford Fairmont with red, fake-leather seats. The car would be about 120° when you got in and the seats would burn your bare skin; the shorts of the mid-1980s were still very short. Nan never inhaled her smoke so we would get all her smoke as well as my parents', who were up in the front. My dad was only there on Fridays and Sundays because he worked on the other days, so it was not so bad on those other days. When my dad was with us, my nan would be in the back with us, so it was quite a tight fit and we three boys had many fights back there on those sweaty vinyl seats. Sitting there, in the smoke and the heat and the traffic, with my brothers' sweaty skin sliding off mine, it was easy to get frustrated. We would only stop fighting when my mother would attempt to hit us while keeping her eyes on the road, doing 60 m.p.h. on the L.I.E. She had a great blind reverse backhand, as did all mothers back in the early '80s.

My grandmother was obsessed with the NY Mets baseball

team and she carried a transistor radio with her everywhere so she could listen to games. As the 1980s progressed the Mets got very good and it became very important for us to be quiet a lot of the time, particularly when the Mets' star player, Daryl Strawberry, was up at the plate. We used to have a spot outside the pool club in the park where we would spend part of the day. We would have barbecues out there on the weekend evenings. My nan hammered a nail into one of the trees in the shade so she could hang her radio on it. That nail stayed there for years and she always had her place to hang the radio. I assume the nail has rusted away by now.

Happy times. The Mets won the World Series in 1986.

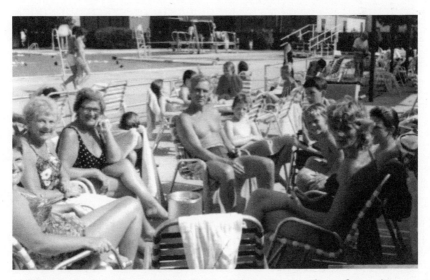

I'm the one hiding under the towel, so I must have been in a mood as I was normally not camera-shy. My nan and Mrs Lennon are on the left and Tommy Kennedy is behind my mother on the right.

My nan's friend from Monaghan, Mrs Lennon, also went out to the pool club with her family. Her kids had all grown up with my mom and her siblings on 160th Street in Flushing. Mrs Lennon's grandson, Tommy Kennedy, was a hero to me as he was a good bit older than me and he took me under his wing. I guess he was the alpha male we had not really known in our house; most of the time our dad was quiet and refined. Tommy was larger than life and full of bravado.

Tommy fancied himself as an underwater swimming champion, and so did my dad, so once they both swam the entire length of the pool underwater, which was pretty impressive as it was quite long. If the underwater swimming competition had no clear winner, my dad's big moment came when Tommy claimed that my dad could not strike him out underhand. In baseball no man likes to be struck out underhand. It is the softball way of pitching, and softball is for girls and fat old men with beer bellies. My father had a wicked way of throwing the ball. He would run up and his arm would do a one-and-a-half turn before he released. He could get some serious speed. Three of my dad's throws struck out Tommy Kennedy underhand.

His ball-throwing style was actually one of the ways I found out that my dad was more Cork than I had given him credit for while growing up. Years later, when I was jogging in Tralee, Co. Kerry, I stumbled upon a bunch of travellers playing a game I had never seen before. I had heard of road bowling because I had lived in Cork for four years, but I had never seen it being played. I knew that only travellers and Cork people still played the game. They let me watch them play and when I saw it I got goosebumps because it took me right back to Mineola Pool Club and I realized that my dad had learned to throw like that in Midleton.

Queens people are no longer allowed to pay for membership at Mineola Pool Club. We stopped going there in 1989 and bought a house in Westhampton before Christmas of that year.

It sounds really posh, but buying the house in the Hamptons was a gamble. The house was on Dune Road in Westhampton and five years earlier the entire area had been destroyed by violent winter storms, mainly Hurricane Gloria. It was still impossible to get anywhere without a four-wheel drive. Houses should never really have been built there in the first place. In fact, there was a court case pending over the area's future. The County of Suffolk was fighting to have the area turned into a state park, and the homeowners were fighting to have the Army Corp of Engineers reclaim the land back from the sea. There was a distinct possibility that it could be deemed unsafe for human habitation. Essentially, my mother gambled that the court case would be won by the homeowners. As a result, my parents got a house (for $80,000) right across the street from the ocean and only an hour and a half from Manhattan.

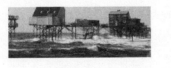 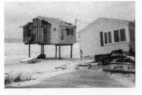

It seems so eerie and dangerous now when I see these pictures. I don't remember it feeling that so much when we were kids.

Those early days there were amazing. It was like a post-apocalyptic scene as half-fallen houses lay open-faced on the beach. Waves broke beneath houses high enough on stilts not to have been washed away yet. The pipes from the septic tanks that had once sat below them hung eerily above the foam. It was a great lesson about the power of the sea.

We would sneak into the abandoned houses all the time. It was fascinating to see how people's lives seemed to have been frozen in time. Often our dad would come with us and we would try to salvage useful things for our own house. The main thing we needed was wood to make walkways over the sand. To this day, when I see a stray bit of wood I immediately assess it for its usefulness.

We became scavengers. It was Westhampton Beyond Thunderdome. We were the Dune Road Warriors, making our house from the wreckage. Sometimes you would see a strange object wash up on the shore like a refrigerator door. The appliances of Dune Road's past were being spat out by the ocean like pistachio shells.

Getting rid of garbage was always a huge issue in our area. In the washed-out years you had to take it to a dump because they could not collect as there was no road to get to the house. Later, after they rebuilt the road and reclaimed the beach, my parents were too cheap to pay for private collection. With all the development going on, my father became obsessed with skips. He had a deep inner skip sense and he would spot them throughout the day. He couldn't drive, so he would bring us in on his scheme. In whispered tones he would say, 'When it's dark we will load up the car with the garbage and you can drive me down the road. I saw a skip there. I will jump out and throw it in fast so no one sees us.' As I got older I stopped coming back so frequently, and Aidan lives with me now and he is still the one who worries about the bins.

Our house was a humble, low-lying bungalow. It sat on the bay side of the road and you could see the most amazing sunsets in the evening during the summer. Its position meant that it sat below the breeze, as the house was sheltered by the high reeds growing out the back. Therefore we were invaders in a land of mosquitoes, and though we never let them win they tormented us nightly and there was more bloodsucking than in a *Twilight* novel. Our evenings were spent in the orange light of the sunset, with the aroma of barbecued cooking and insect repellant in the air.

There was a good crew of people in their early thirties who played volleyball on the beach every weekend. None of them had kids yet and they welcomed us into their circle on the beach. At fourteen I was just about old enough to make up an even number to play a game, and my dad was just about young enough to do the same. I can actually remember the day they let me play for the first time. I did not believe them at first, but then they were waiting for me to come on the court. I would spend the next six summers of my life wanting to be on that court as much as I could. It is still one of my favourite things to do in the world, to play beach volleyball.

Me, Michael John and Aidan absolutely idolized those guys. I would say they had a serious influence on us growing up because they were very different from the type of people we grew up with in Queens. They were all professional people from the city and maybe they were more sophisticated. I just remember that I loved trying to impress them. I think they found us very entertaining because we were pretty wild kids and liked to mess around. All those guys loved to joke around too and pass on the knowledge of the area to us since they had been coming out there forever.

Stu was one of the guys on the beach and he loved to joke around. One day I remember becoming very frustrated over something on the court. I argued to the point of my frustration boiling over and I had a hissy fit and walked off the court. I could hear Stu shouting as I walked away, 'Why don't you go home and shave your goatee and put a dress on!' I had a goatee that day – which must have been comical as I was never a very hairy guy, and it must have taken me a month to grow enough hair for anyone even to be able to see it. So I had to walk over the dunes with the sense that everyone was laughing at me and I had just made an ass of myself.

I wanted to just turn back, but my pride would not let me. I was back in the house, kicking and screaming to myself, so pissed off at myself for losing my head, and then it hit me. I went to the bathroom and shaved off my goatee. I went to the linen closet and wrapped a sheet around my chest like a summer dress and walked back over to the beach. It was the only way I could go back. I was admitting that I was an asshole but also that I had a sense of humour. It was like a penance for messers. They were all laughing hard at that one. Those were very happy summers.

Throughout all those years my dad would just sit on the beach for hours and stare out at the sea, lost deep in his thoughts. All our lives we would come across our father lost in thought. It often seemed his life was elsewhere. He loved telling us that the ocean was mighty. He loved telling our friends who would come out that it was all about the ocean. Most of our friends' dads talked about cars and the NY Mets, but my dad wanted to know how the ocean made you feel.

7

When I was a kid I believed every one of my dad's stories. So far as I was concerned he was pretty famous when he was younger. I did not know much else about his life other than his career as an actor and a model; he had been in the British Army and had lived in Midleton, Co. Cork, during World War II. Sometimes he would be watching TV and would recognize someone he knew from his past. One I always remember was Robert Shaw from *Jaws*. *Jaws* was a big movie

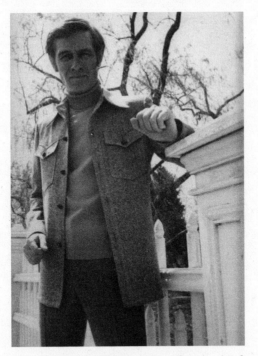

One of my dad's final modelling jobs after he had moved back to New York.

in our hood and the fact that my dad knew somebody from it was pretty cool. I can't remember some of the other claims he made, but I remember finding an old modelling photo of his which included all the clients of an agency he was with at the time. His picture was very close to Cybill Shepherd's, and at the time she was in *Moonlighting* with Bruce Willis. She was incredibly beautiful and I was very impressed.

I knew that my dad had been in a movie or two and had done a few ads, including a Blue Nun advert that used to run on RTÉ. Years later, when I met my cousins in Midleton, they would all say to me, 'Red or White, darling? BLUE!' That was my dad's line in the commercial. But when we were kids the only movie that mattered to us was *The Day of the Triffids*. It was not a big movie by any means, but my dad had a proper scene in it. It's a pretty silly horror B-movie, but we had a copy of the videotape when we were kids. Of course it was my cousin Ira who got it for us. I think it was as important for him to keep the legend of my dad going as it was for us. Up until he sourced a copy, I only had Ira's word for it that my dad had a lot of lines. Ira always said my dad was a blind pilot trying to land the plane. 'Mayday! Mayday!' Ira would always say.

Then we got the movie and we could watch it all the time. We would rewind back to the beginning of his scene and watch it over and over. 'Mayday! Mayday! Please talk us down.' It seemed like a massive scene when we were kids. I watch it now and I think it's quite short, but we were just in awe back then. He has this extra-long close-up, right at the end of the scene, which appeared to last for ages. We thought this was the coolest thing. It took me years to find anyone who had ever heard of the film *The Day of the Triffids*, but I would show it to my friends when they came over.

All my friends loved my dad. They loved his accent, and

he would always tell them ghost stories. He was great at doing Dracula stories. They would always begin with him saying slowly, 'It was a daaarrk, daarrrk night . . .' I can still picture a large group of us, sitting in the living room one early evening while my dad was telling one of his stories, and how mesmerized we were by it. He was doing it differently on this particular night and he never got to the actual Dracula story because after a five-minute intro of slow 'daaarrk, daarrrk nights' and wind noises, he shouted something really loudly and we all jumped, completely startled. It was great. He was a great performer for my friends. It's cool when you are young and the young girls that you are beginning to take notice of tell you that your dad is cool. 'Did you know that Des's dad was a model?' 'Did you know that Des's dad was in a movie?'

When we were kids, there wasn't much to dislike about my dad, but he didn't really have much authority in the house. The truth was, if our family was a company my mother was the managing director and my dad just did the PR. If it had been left to him, we would have looked amazing but we would have been starving. One of the few things I can remember my dad really caring about was that we didn't get fat. 'If you keep eating those cookies you will end up being as fat as a house.'

My mother was the boss. We were never even allowed to ask my dad for permission to do things. If we did, knowing that my mother would say no afterwards, she would say, 'You know that's not the way it works in this house.' He never even had a driver's licence. This added to his dependence on my mother and to our view of him as not being much of an authority figure.

To us, our dad was just cool and fun. He never gave me a hard time about school or homework. He just encouraged us to do well in sports and he hated it when we spoke like real Queens kids. He never really corrected us, but he would just tell us we sounded rough. My mother was very Catholic and was adamant that we go to Mass every Sunday. My father didn't mind. He always fell asleep at Mass but would wake up for the songs because he loved to sing. My mother hated the singing and once wrote a letter to Monsignor Fogarty complaining that the 'Our Father' was not a song and should not be sung at Mass. It was a good example of how different they were from each other.

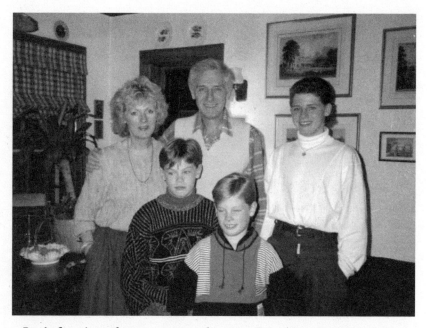

Let's face it, puberty was cruel to me. I woke up one morning and this afro was on top of my head where once my wavy hair had been. And look at the style. It must have been in the one-week window when MC Hammer was cool; Hammer-time was a lonely time for me. What was I thinking, with those trousers up to my nipples and the turtleneck with the medallion? I actually thought that made me look cool. It turns out it made me look like a young lesbian.

Up until I hit puberty, most of the time I just saw my dad as a really cool guy. I was too young to be aware that he was not the authority figure. He was just the guy I always wanted to impress. He was the guy I wanted to see watching me do things. 'Dad, watch me dive off the diving board.' 'Dad, count how long I can stay under water.' 'Dad, listen to me do the beat box.' He was myself and my brothers' hero.

But it all changed when I became a teenager. I developed a desire to challenge my dad's authority. I went from thinking my parents were the coolest people on the planet to thinking they were the dumbest people to walk the face of the earth. I think Mark Twain said it best when he said, 'When I was a boy of fourteen, my father was so ignorant I could hardly stand to have the old man around. But when I got to be twenty-one, I was astonished by how much he'd learned in seven years.'

I had entered my period of rebellion and my brothers would enter that period at two-year intervals behind me. We expressed it by making fun of my father all the time.

When our dad went from being the only person we wanted to impress, he became the butt of our jokes and our attempts to impress each other. We were like diehard fans who turn on their idols with a vengeance. We had outgrown his style. He was not cool anymore. I know a lot of people go through that phase, but I think for us a few things were different. First, we were all like our dad, in that much of what we did in the house was a performance. Second, our dad let us make fun of him with minimal retribution. And finally, most people do not have a dad who was in a cheesy 1960s British movie like *The Day of the Triffids*.

It was one of my running jokes for a while. Any time my dad would get pissed off at me for something and raise his voice, I would say in a British accent, 'MAYDAY, MAYDAY.

Please talk us down.' Or if he shouted up the stairs at me, 'Desmond, get down these stairs right this minute!' I would say, 'PLEASE TALK US DOWN, MAYDAY, MAYDAY! THERE IS STILL NO REPLY, SIR.' These were his lines from the movie. My brothers and I thought we were being so funny when we did that over the years.

Though I was not aware of it at the time, I suppose we were actually making fun of the fact that often he wasn't present, either in mind or body. He always forgot people's names and very often would fall asleep on the bus and wake up out in New Hyde Park, Long Island. He would call up, all panicked, 'I fell asleep, man. Tell your mother when she gets home that I am out in New Hyde Park.' You could often hear him cursing to himself as he hung up the phone. In the end we used to insult each other by saying, 'You're just like Dad!'

It was when I was in my teens that I became convinced that my dad was a spoofer. And for a large part of my life I went on believing that. 'Never let the truth get in the way of a good story' was definitely something he believed. His life story was always confusing to us anyway. So many of his memories had overlapping timelines. Things didn't add up. It was easy for us to believe that he was just making up a lot of his past.

Not only did I think that his stories were bullshit, but I also thought he had used his charm to get through life and that he was actually not a very smart man. He was an incredibly nice man in my eyes, but I felt he had used his niceness to hide the fact that he was inherently silly. I don't know where this thought came from originally. I guess I shouldn't be too hard on myself, because there were often times when he would try to show off, just to fit in, and would talk about things he knew nothing about, which would kind of embarrass me. But now I know that was not because he was stupid, he was just too proud or too desperate to be liked not to put in his two cents' worth on every subject.

He always found a way to connect himself to someone, wherever they were from. It was usually through sports. If someone was from India he would talk about cricket. If someone was from Argentina he would talk about Diego Maradona. Within a minute of meeting someone he would always ask, 'Where are you from, my friend?' After a while we knew that if they were from India he was going to talk about some cricketer called Singh, and he would then say, 'Gandhi was a great man!' He would sometimes botch it up though, give himself away in small ways – things like calling over a waiter with a commanding '*Signor!*' when the restaurant was Greek.

His worst blunder though came in Burberrys when Liam Gallagher from Oasis came into the store. My father was assigned to make sure everything was all right for him. Of course my father did not know who he was, so his first question was, 'Where are you from, my friend?' When Gallagher said, 'Manchester,' my father said, 'Manchester United are an amazing team.' Gallagher replied, 'I am a City fan, I fuckin' hate Man United.' And walked away.

We really went to town on him when I discovered he had been secretly watching porn on the TV. This happened after my mother kindly but unwittingly laid on free hardcore porn for us. She had got our cousin Teddy to get us an illegal cable box, which was then all the rage in Queens. It meant that we paid for basic cable service, but we got all of the channels all of the time, including the pay-per-view movie channels, so we could watch all the latest releases for free. That is really why my mother wanted it, so she could watch movies when repeats of *Murder, She Wrote* weren't on.

She did not realize that there was a pay-per-view movie channel called the Spice Network that showed hotel-room standard porn 24/7. This stuff was not the French soft porn we used to have to trawl the TV guide to find. This was full-on porn-star porn all the time. Well, this was a gift for us three boys who had just entered the height of our masturbatory prowess. I was sixteen and was in need of porn for at least three to four years. My brother Michael John was fourteen and was definitely on the hunt, and Aidan was just entering the realm of self-help.

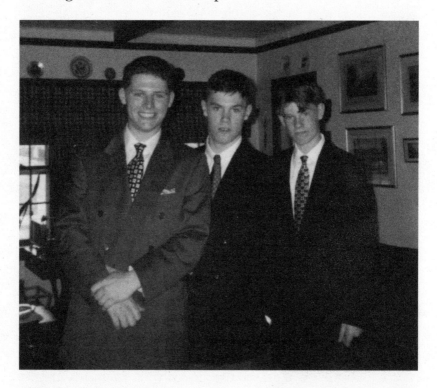

Porn was a rare thing to come across in the early 1990s. It's not like now, when you can find it on the internet. We watched it all the time. But we assumed we were the only ones in the house watching it.

One day I came home at one o'clock in the morning and I

caught my dad watching the Spice Network. Now when I say I had caught him, he was actually watching Channel 62, the Japanese channel which was one channel down from Spice. It's important to understand that until the day he died my father did not know how to use the remote control; he called it the 'flicker'. He called it that because the only thing he knew was flicking through the channels with the arrow keys. He never figured out that you could just press two number buttons one after the other. He would have thought that going from 5 to 85 in one go was magic. Watching TV with my dad was seriously annoying, as getting from one channel to another involved him flicking through all the channels in between. Maybe in 1990s Ireland it wasn't annoying to Flick, Flick, BOOM – all the channels – but we had 130 of them.

However, this became a big problem for my dad when I walked in unexpectedly. He must have thought I was upstairs in bed when in fact I had been across the street getting drunk in another kid's basement. So I took him by surprise and he was quick enough on the draw to only flick one channel down. Therefore he had to sit confidently in front of a period Japanese soap opera with no subtitles that he had no business watching whatsoever. I knew straight away what he was doing. I watched Spice every day and I knew very well that the Japanese channel was one down. He was screwed either way, because 64 was the Arab channel.

I was willing to give my dad a chance to keep his dignity, so I let him come up with an excuse. I asked him, 'What are you doing watching the Japanese channel?' All he could think of to say was, 'Well, they come into Burberrys so I thought I'd watch what they watch.'

It is actually really funny when your dad appears to be in trouble in front of you, and it was too funny not to tell my brothers. For a long time after that we would sometimes put on Japanese accents and ask my father if he wanted to watch TV with us. 'Ooooh, Michaelson, very good soap opera on today. Flicky, Flicky 62 for you. But oh be very careful do not a flicky flicky too faa. Sixty-three verrrry diiirty.' It was silly and, until my mother saw the routine about it in the stage show, she never knew why we used to do that.

8

One of the running jokes in our family was doing my dad's accent and saying, 'I am going to study the rules of the road and take the test this year.' He was always going on about it. Actually, because he couldn't drive I don't have that many memories of just being with my dad on my own when I was young.

One day, about six years before he died, we were driving down 188th Street by Peck Park and I asked him why he never learned to drive. Then I asked him when was the last time he had actually even tried to drive. He told me he could hardly remember. It was not a busy time of day so I pulled over and told him he should give it a go right that minute. For some reason he said yes; he must have been in a very good mood. It's a strange thing to teach your dad to drive. It's not meant to happen that way; it is supposed to be the other way around.

The first thing he did was to ask me where the clutch was. Now this will tell you how clueless he was because he had been driving with my mother in America since 1976 and had never figured out that in an automatic transmission there is no clutch. My mother never drove a manual transmission in her life, so there had been no time in their life together when he could even have heard mention of the clutch. So I told him there was no clutch and that it was the same as going on the bumper cars. Of course he had never gone on the bumper cars with us because of his back, but I think he got the gist of what I was trying to say.

So he got behind the wheel and made the usual mistake of putting his left foot on the brake. I told him to use just the right foot, and away we went up the hill on 188th Street, two blocks from our house. He was not bad. The best moment was when he said, almost childlike, 'Holy shit, man, I am bloody driving!'

He panicked a bit as we came up to the stop sign at our corner, where he stopped and we swapped places so I could park the car, but he had done well. He said he was going to learn the rules of the road so he could drive in retirement and not have to rely on my mother. But of course he didn't.

When my mother went through his stuff after he died, she found three copies of the rules of the road study manual in his drawer.

My father wasn't a total pushover and we had some proper clashes during those turbulent teenage years, but later on I wondered why he allowed us to make fun of him as much as we did. At times our dinners became like a sketch show, all based on us doing impersonations of my dad. As an adult I thought back to those times and wondered why my dad had never stood up and properly let us know that he had had enough. A lot of it was good fun, but more of it was disrespectful. I sometimes wished when I got older that he had slammed his fist on the table and let us know who was the boss.

In the house it was all about our performance, and my dad took a lot of slagging; but outside the house it was a different matter because there were other people observing us. My father's favourite thing to say to us was, 'Don't make a scene.' He was essentially a very quiet man in the very loud world of New York children with a very loud New York wife. My mother loved making a scene. It was in drama that she functioned best. It's quite funny that a man who desired the spotlight much of the time hated the drama of everyday life. My mother hated the spotlight, but she loved the drama. This was also unfortunate for my dad, because he hated sudden loud noises in the house and would often jump when we were shouting or knocked something over.

We grew up with the language of chaos. My mother described everything as a disaster. Now we do. I can hear it when my brothers say it nowadays. Of course, out of our New York mouths it sounds like, 'Dis is a *disasta*!' A long line at customs: Dis is a *disasta*. Waiter taking too long to bring the food: What a *disasta*. Ordering a taxi that takes too long to arrive: Dis is a *disasta*.

I too always describe the most basic problems as a disaster. For example, if I ended up in traffic I would say, 'This is a disaster!' It's not the right word to use, because an earthquake is a disaster; traffic is a minor inconvenience. I was never really aware of how frequently I said things were a disaster. One day, while I was making a documentary, the director Mike Casey said to me, 'I realize now that you just use that word in a specific way. For a while I thought you genuinely viewed things as disasters, but now I know it's just the way you describe things.' It came to me that he had been thinking until then that my radar of how serious a situation is was quite irrational.

The strange thing is that we never viewed the big things as *disastas* at all. I don't think anyone once described my dad getting sick as a *disasta*. I can hardly remember my mom getting breast cancer because she wouldn't let us know how it was going. In fact, if you ever asked my mother how she was around that time, she would tell you it was nothing. It certainly was not a *disasta*. Not like getting parking at North Shore Hospital on her way in to treatment. 'Gawd, what a *disasta*!'

My father always tried to remain calm. He was not great at anything confrontational. That's why he always said things like 'Don't make a scene'; or maybe it was because we were always making scenes. Us boys made the scenes that hyper kids make when they fight in public, and my mother made the scenes that battleaxe women make when they are trying to get deals or are fighting against car dealers who are trying to pull a fast one. Perhaps my dad did not like us making scenes because he was not in them. Maybe he was such an actor he would have preferred to be the one making the scene, because then he would be the star of it.

I sometimes wonder if I am wrong about feeling that I had a very passive father, so while writing this book I asked my mother what she thought. She told me that my dad never really wanted to be our father as much as he wanted to be our friend. He was too worried that if he was tough on us we would reject him. He just wanted us to love him, which frustrated my mother. I never really knew that, but she often felt that it was her versus all the men in the house. She does have a tendency to see herself as the victim, so I take that with a pinch of salt, but she certainly always had to be the bad cop. The problem was, my dad was not even playing the good cop; he wasn't being a cop at all. He was just waiting for us to get out of the interrogation room so he could play some more. He left the police work to her.

If I were to say what kind of cop my mother was, I would say she was like Mel Gibson in *Lethal Weapon*. She got the job done but she had a pretty crazy way of going about it. She had everyone around her on edge all the time. But she had learned to fuel herself with anxiety because anxiety was all she ever really knew while growing up. This is not really my mother's story, but it is important to know that she had a really tough childhood, which I found out about quite late in life. My grandmother was one of the most loving women I could have known in my lifetime, but after she died (in 1998) I found out that my grandparents had been terrible alcoholics and my mother and her siblings had had to deal with the unpredictability of that throughout all their childhood. My mother told me she often had to pull her mother out of the local bars and would have to deal with my grandmother's harsh and shame-filled rants when she was boozed up.

In my show I joke that my mother was American but was raised in the proper Irish way, in that she was raised by alcoholics. People always laugh, both in Ireland and in the UK. I know that why they laugh is because of the way I phrase it, but I always think that it should not be funny. It is kind of darkly humorous to know that so many people in the crowd are laughing from pure identification. They are thinking, 'Is there any other way to be raised? I thought one of your parents being an alky was part of it. That's how it works: most of the time your parents are angry and every now and then they come home happy at one in the morning and you begin to associate affection with the smell of chips!'

We did not grow up around booze, so that image comes more from the family life I saw when I was staying with friends in Ireland after I moved there to go to boarding school when I was fourteen. I witnessed those Dr Jekyll and Mr Hyde parents many times. But my mother was not an observer of that life, she was an active participant. There are so many stories of what she had to go through. She used to hate going to Gaelic Park with Michael John and Aidan when they got into playing Gaelic football in the Bronx when they grew a bit older. Gaelic Park was a very emotional place for her because she could remember spending all day Sunday there when she was a girl, watching Gaelic football in the heat and then having to drag her parents out of the bar and carry them to the subway and get them all the way back to Queens.

When I found out about all this I was kind of impressed with what she had had to get through. She had survived The War of the Alcoholic Home. She had survived the stress and the uncertainty. She survived that war by developing the survival skills of wartime. She had found a way of coping in this very turbulent situation when she should have just been being a kid and worrying about playing and doing homework. That could not have been easy.

I always say that it is amazing my mother survived it. The fact that she had to develop those wartime skills to get through it was tremendous and I commend her for developing them. It was just unfortunate for myself and my brothers that she chose to use the same skills in *peacetime* and brought a little bit of that war home to the sober Bishop household. There was no need for all that drama, but that was all she knew. Crisis management was her strong point, so she needed to create a crisis in order to manage it. This meant that as kids we grew up with an enormous amount of anxiety without there really being that much to be anxious about.

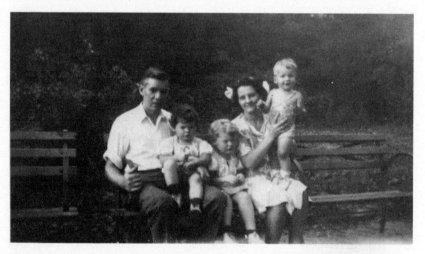

My mother's family enjoying Kissena Park in the mid-1940s.
From the left: her father John O'Hare ('Pop Pop'), my Aunt
Mary, my mom, my nan Peggy O'Hare and my Uncle Jack.
There were still two more to come – my Uncle Kev and my
Aunt Peggy.

If you want further evidence of how this manifested itself in our lives, I can tell you about times when my dad would have his blowouts. When I say a 'blowout' I just mean when my father would blow his fuse. He rarely did so, but when he did it was pretty strong. He would often ask to be let out of the car wherever we were.

'Stop the car, Eileen! Stop the car, now!'

Big drama. My father would get out of the car and walk away. It was not a really cool thing to do and my mother would be seriously panicked. After an hour or so, if my dad had not come home my mother would pack me in the car and drive around to the local bars, looking for him. She would send me in to take a peak to see if he was in there. I would have thought it was cool if he was in one of them. Not realizing that he had had a drink problem, I would not have thought it at all strange when I was small if my dad had decided to have a beer in a local bar. That's what grown-ups did.

Of course we would not find him because he was always just walking around Kissena or Peck Park, or he would just go for a haircut or something to cool down. But my mother's reflex was to go back to that place of terror.

Actually that is one other really interesting thing about my dad. Any time he 'blew his stack', which was his way of describing it, within a day or two he would always apologize to us. He might also say, 'Hey, Dessie Doodle, I am sorry I lost my cool, man!' It was always pretty cool that he would do that.

One final thing I've realized about my parents as I work on this book. When I go through all the family photographs, I notice there are hardly any of us with my mother. That is because she was taking them all. She was the director. She was the one behind the scenes. Perhaps she should have let herself take part more. Perhaps my dad should have insisted on getting her in. It just became the way it was. That was the role she played. She did not have time to horse around, because the whole production was resting on her shoulders. It had been since she was just a girl.

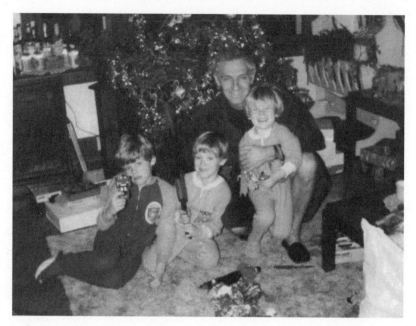

Once again it's my mother taking the picture. All the photos with her in them were taken really badly. My father was made for one side of the lens only and was always terrible with gadgets. I loved that Transformer.

9

The weird thing that happened to me in the early days of my father's illness was realizing just how much I was like my mother. Though I had followed in my father's footsteps in so many other ways, my personality was much more like my mother's. I have a short fuse, like her, and I am not very patient. In the past, my mother would have been the one to take charge in a family crisis like this, but she was not really able to take charge in that first week after my dad's diagnosis. My brother Michael John and I had to have all the chats and relay the information to my mother and hide most of it from my father.

Suddenly the children were in charge. And I was also into being in charge. I even noticed that once or twice in the first day or two I would get annoyed when people did not want to do things my way. It had nothing to do with what was best for my father and everything to do with me being right. I remember actually thinking to myself: *'I AM MY MOTHER!'*

Even when he moved into a nicer room after his initial assessments were over, my father was still not sleeping well. I think it was after his first day of chemo that he asked me quite innocently if he could have a sleeping tablet. I rang for the nurse and I asked her if my father could have one. She told us that she had to ask the doctor first. That was not much of a big deal, but for some reason they could not find a doctor who could answer that question for my dad. It probably should not have been that much of a drama, but it was late and my father was pushing us to leave because he was feeling bad that we had been there all day. My mother on the other hand would not go until I had secured a sleeping pill for my father. Suddenly it was up to me to try and get this pill for him.

Life goes on in the hospital and, of course, to the nurse there was nothing urgent about the situation. I called again fifteen minutes later and she had still not got an answer for us. The long day and my mother's worry were not helping my ability to deal with my growing frustration and I was losing patience big time. In fact the frustration of everything that had gone on in the last few days was building up in me, along with the responsibility of getting this pill for him, no matter what. Of course my dad was trying to say that it was not important, but it was not even about him anymore. It was all about the fact that this was ridiculous. It was not a big deal and I was moving beyond any rational reaction to the delay in getting an answer to my request.

In the end the nurse came back with a negative response: the doctor had said my father could not have a sleeping pill. My mother made the noises that she makes when she is not happy with the situation. I then got a little upset with the nurse about why it took so long to find out such a simple thing. I was making a scene and my father hated that. He was probably thinking: 'Oh my god, he's become Eileen. The metamorphosis is complete!'

My dad must have felt compelled (as he had done for most of his life) to try and chill out the situation. How he did it was quite funny. I did not really see it as such at the time, because I was quite worked up. He turned to me in front of everyone and said, 'Look, Des, it's all right, if I don't get a sleeping pill, I won't lose any sleep over it!'

Everyone laughed. I kind of laughed too but I was annoyed that he was undermining my attempt to push for him in the hospital. It was as if, only a few days into my newfound authority in the family, my new parent/son was undermining my authority as I had once done his. Here was me back in NY, cancelling all my shows, so I could look after my dad and pay him back for looking after me as a child. And he was trying to pay me back for being a smart ass when I was a teenager.

This might be the most light-hearted and quickest account of a father's alcoholism you will ever read. My father was sober in my lifetime and, except for one slip, I was never aware of my dad being drunk. I did not even know he was in AA until I was thirteen years old. I knew this because all my dad's friends were in AA and they used to come over on New Year's Eve. One of them, John Gilholey, used to bring his daughter over. Of course, as the years went by, we hit puberty, and one New Year's Eve Tracy Gilholey was the first girl I properly made out with. We were up in the attic while they were downstairs.

After that night we got to chatting on the phone and I asked her how our dads knew each other and she said it was probably from AA. This was a total shock to me. In fact I did not believe it until I found my dad's copy of the AA book, *Twenty-Four Hours a Day*, and it said: 'Church on the Hill AA Group'. All my life my parents would mention Church on the Hill. Every Monday and Saturday my dad would go there. Eventually it just became 'The Hill'. I am sure we even said to my dad, 'Are you going to The Hill?' Until I found this out I just thought it was weird that my parents didn't drink.

My dad had one slip, and I thought it was cool. There was an empty bottle of wine downstairs and my dad was asleep on the couch. I was delighted because I thought it was so funny. My mother was not delighted, obviously, but she had more back story than I did. She herself had given up booze when she got pregnant with me and she never drank again. She saw herself as having a problem, but she was not a member of AA.

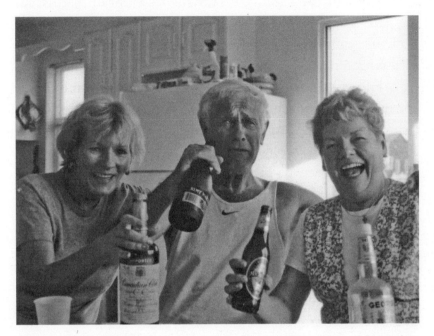

My parents with my Aunt Mary out in the Hamptons. I love this picture because none of them drank anymore at this time and they were pretending to be drunk. Look how happy they are – even pretending works!

So I don't know that much about my dad's drinking. I know that when he moved to London from East Sussex in his mid-twenties, booze quickly became a huge part of his life. He was connected to a big drinking scene in which most of the actors and models drank all day. He was actually sober when he moved to New York in 1969 to work for the Ford Modelling Agency. My parents met even before he had a place to live; they met at an advertising agency party to welcome the London models to New York. He was not drinking in those early days and my mother went to some AA meetings with him, as she was concerned about her own drinking problems.

By the time my parents were living together in Manhattan my dad's back problems had taken a very bad turn. He got back into drinking and developed a fondness for painkillers. As a result he began to miss jobs and Ford was not too happy with him. One day my mother had to call an ambulance because my father was immobilized by pain. He ended up in Bellevue Hospital and had to have another operation. His convalescence was long and he moved in with my grand-mother in Queens while he was recovering. She was very good to him at that time and this was one of the reasons why he was so incredibly fond of her. By the time he recovered, he found that the work had dried up. His only thought was to move back to London and pick up where he had left off. My mother agreed to go with him.

It was a good move and he began to get loads of work in and around 1971. My parents lived in Putney and my mother enjoyed the London life. Then, some time in 1972, Nevs, the model agency that was looking after him, organized for him to move to Düsseldorf in Germany, where there was much money to be made. My mother speaks fondly of this time as they had an amazing flat full of antiques, she had her own job and Dad was making loads of money. My father's drink-ing was the only source of tension in the relationship, and things came to a head when my father got a job modelling for a Pushkin Vodka advertising campaign, which meant he would be in Iceland for two months. My mother told him she would not stay in Germany on her own for that long. She flew back to New York the following day and began working in her brother Jack's bar, called the Rub a Dub Pub, in Middle Village in Queens. My dad went to Iceland.

Months passed and one day my mother got a call from my dad's friend, the publican Eamon Doran, to say that there was someone in town who wanted to talk to her. It was my dad and he told her he was getting a taxi to Queens to see her. That night he told her he wanted to marry her. He got what he wanted, and within two months – in May 1973 – they got married and set up home in an apartment in Queens.

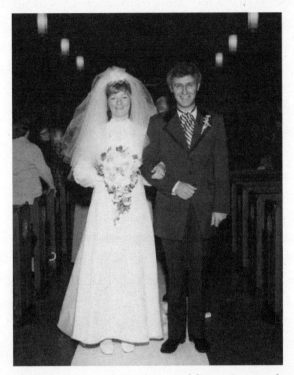

My dad was never crazy about his wedding pictures because he had a brutal hangover and always thought he looked terrible.

Booze was still a source of tension, and after an argument (about my mother's drinking, oddly enough) my father decided to leave and go to Ireland. I don't know why he decided to do that, but it was quite a dramatic move. My mother was left on her own and had to get rid of the apartment and move home.

She thought that was the end of things and that she would never hear from him again, but eventually he called from London and asked her to move there to be with him, and she agreed. They moved into a place my mother remembers as 'the Irish house', where there were a lot of Irish actors. It was definitely not the best place to be living if booze was causing problems in your life.

Later, Nevs organized an apartment for them on Markham Square, off the King's Road in Chelsea. They had a great life. My mother loved her job, working for the Australian company Rio Tinto. Dad got good modelling work and he made a lot of money.

After they moved back to London, I know that my dad was in and out of AA. My mother was also still drinking. When her father died in January 1975, she made a vow to the Blessed Mother, with whom she feels a great connection, that if she got pregnant she would never drink again. At that stage she had been trying to conceive for a while and she was beginning to panic. She got pregnant soon afterwards, and she never drank again. She liked to joke that I might be the reincarnation of her father. I know that in the end my mother gave my father an ultimatum about his drinking because she was not going to raise her child in a house of booze. She had been raised in a house like that, and she was not going to repeat it.

She gave her mother an ultimatum, too. My nan sailed to London in 1975. She got off the boat, stinking of booze, and my mother was devastated because she had been sober for a while before that. She told her mother that she could have nothing to do with her children if she continued to drink. My mother had pretty much had it with the negative effects of booze in her life. I never saw my nan drunk and I never knew she was an alcoholic until I was much older. My mother liked keeping even the mention of booze as far away as possible from us. She did not want us to end up that way. She fought hard and failed, but God loves a trier.

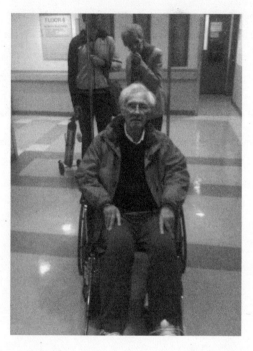

Journal, 16 November 2009, Flushing, Queens, 6.39 a.m.

I had been looking forward to getting some time to write down some of the powerful things that have happened, but the reality of the situation came crashing down on me in the last few hours. I woke up to the sound of my father moaning in the bathroom. He had not made it to the toilet and had had an accident. When I walked in he was just sitting there, embarrassed, and I have to say for a few seconds I just looked on in shock.

There was shit on the floor and all over his legs. My
mother woke up and we quickly went about dealing with
the situation. His pyjamas were badly soiled, but we just
got on with it. The smell was terrible, but I did not gag
because I did not want him to realize how disgusting it
was as I didn't want him to feel even more uncomfortable.

The minute you begin the clean-up, something changes
and it does not really seem like a big deal. The yellow
water, the stained cloth and what was left on his leg no
longer seemed dirty. The acceptance comes so rapidly.
You don't give it a thought as you wring the cloth and
yellow water streams across your hand. The more yellow
the water becomes, the better, because you want him to
get clean. I wanted to make him feel fresh again. I rubbed
his swollen legs down, and they were so swollen I just
wanted him to let go and not bother fighting.

I tried to make him laugh by asking him if he realized
shit was yellow. As I wiped his bum I reminded him that
only a few years ago I had joked that one day I would
be wiping his ass – I had just not expected it to come so
soon.

Most of all, though, I just felt sorry for him. He was so
helpless on the toilet, speaking about how embarrassed
he felt. He was not a fan of the jokes as he was normally
so terribly private about this type of stuff. 'Oh come
on, man, please! This is not funny!' I wished he was
not embarrassed around me. I just wondered if he was
thinking how it had got to this point so fast. He seemed
so helpless, it was hard to bear.

We got him back to the bed, clean and smelling fresh.
We joked about cockney slang and before he lay down he
sang some of the cockney songs he wrote for his musical.
Then he reminded me that it was he who wrote it, as if

he had invented cockney slang himself. His vanity had returned, and I could rest easy.

Journal, 17 November 2009, Flushing, Queens, 10.03 a.m.

Another morning, and we have developed a routine. Wake up, check in with my dad and then begin trying to motivate my dad to eat. He is doing pretty good on that front, but I can tell he does not enjoy it. His appetite has not come back at all and he told me he would gladly not eat for the entire day.

It is Mom's birthday today and she really did not want to make a fuss. I did buy her a card and some scratch cards, which I think she enjoyed getting, but she cried when reading the cards. For definite, she is finding this much harder than the rest of us. The mood swings can be hard to deal with, but, to her and our credit, we have been doing pretty good at keeping the communication very open. Yesterday it got pretty intense and an argument between myself and Aidan and my mother culminated in her admitting that she was afraid. I had never heard my mother say those words.

You begin to feel as if you're living two lives. There is the life upstairs with my father, which is overflowing with love, service and motivation. There are no barriers up there. We have had wonderful discussions about the acceptance of death, the dismissal of regret and buckets of indulgence in nostalgia. It is an affectionate life upstairs, where hugs and back-stroking are in large supply. I have lain down next to him for ages, with his hand in my hand in the most natural way. Despite the horror of what is happening, there is something so beautiful developing as a result.

Then there is the life downstairs. Here there are no hidden facts to soften the blow. Down below is the harsh reality of care. There is the cold truth of organization, health insurance, information and preparation. Every time the phone rings there is hope, dread, fear and annoyance.

Down below there is my mother about to lose the only life she has ever known, or at least a life that has existed long enough to have erased the memory of what had been before. I find it frustrating that she chooses to hold on to miracles as her way of coping. She rejects what is going on upstairs as an admission of defeat. She can't engage with it at all. I try to bring her in but she keeps her ear cocked for a noise from the room, like a dog during a thunderstorm, and, given any chance, she heads away into her safety zone of responsibility and care. She pretends that she has been open with Dad about things, but I know she hasn't.

It is tough because I want to help them both equally, but it was easier to deal with her in those first few days when she was helpless and vulnerable. Now she is determined to organize everything every minute of the day. I know it helps her to be busy and to feel like she is doing everything she can, but sometimes it just leaves you feeling a bit cold.

Journal, 21 November 2009, Flushing, Queens

Things have settled down. My father has rekindled his interest in watching the English Premiership all through Saturday. There is nothing immediate. My dad seems stable. Chemo does not start again for nine days and all the prescriptions are filled. This helps my mother to relax, which helps everyone else to unwind. We have moved away from the intense emotions of the last few weeks. The accidents have stopped and there is no more drama.

Yesterday I saw such a lovely thing. My father had befriended a young girl from the house next door. Her name is Jenny and she moved here from China when she was only a baby. Sometime in the early years of her life in Flushing herself and my dad developed a friendship. I believe they made a snowman during one of the snowstorms. Over the years since they have become quite close and she has been dying to get in and see him since she heard he was ill.

She came in yesterday with the cutest card that she had made herself, with all her own messages of support and motivation. There was a body-builder cut out of a magazine and she had written 'You are strong'. The card was huge and pink and full of little cut-outs and drawings she did herself. In big letters it said 'I LOVE YOU'.

She came in and they hugged. My father held her for ages and said, 'My little friend, Jenny.' It really made me cry.

When my dad first got sick I decided to keep a journal. That is where these journal entries and the ones in Part Three come from. It can be hard to remember how you feel at these intense moments and I wanted to have something to remind me. But looking back on them, I've realized that the entries come to a sudden stop. There are about ten for the first six weeks of my dad being sick, and then only two more for the following three months.

Originally I thought that maybe this was because he began to feel better and we had got into a routine, but my mother reminded me that it was around then that I bought a box set of the HBO series *The Wire*. *The Wire* took over our lives more than cancer did. So did street language – and, of course, the way Senator Clay Davis says, 'SHEEEEIIIIITTTT.' Now, for those who have not seen *The Wire* this won't mean much, but for us it completely took us away from what was going on. I watched every single episode with my mother and father. My mother told me that at that time she began to organize the day so we could just sit down and watch three uninterrupted episodes.

When I hear the opening song now, I just think of that time. When I hear the music that finishes an episode I just think of us looking at each other and saying, 'Will we go for one more?' The opening song has a repeated line, about putting the devil down in the hole. We heard that song four or five times a day. After a few weeks my dad and I would be having breakfast and he would look up at me and say, 'You wanna go down in the hole?' That was his way of asking if we could watch some of *The Wire*. It's all we thought about for nearly eight weeks; we did not think about cancer: we put that devil way down in the hole.

12

My dad was the general manager of the Burberrys flagship store on East 57th Street for most of my life. Essentially he was just a store manager, but it seemed a lot more prestigious because it was a big store with a famous name, and it was on a street that at one stage had the most expensive rent on the planet.

People are very familiar with Burberrys today, but it was not that way when we were growing up. This was before the Burberry check became the national flag of the British degenerate. Young people did not really know about Burberrys, so it was not that exciting to tell people what my dad did. My friends' parents used to care though, particularly the dads; in the 1980s the Burberry trenchcoat was a must-have for a Manhattan businessman. Most of my friends' dads were tradesmen or cops, but even the cops used to love showing off to their friends the fact that they had some Burberry which was really out of their price range.

Some of the dads worked on Wall Street, however, and they were really big fans of the discounts my dad could get for them. I really only became aware of that when I got a bit older, but still when I meet some of them when I am back in Queens they will always say they think of my dad when they wear the raincoat or the sweater he got for them at a discount. Not that I am promoting Burberrys; but it has to be said, the quality is fantastic. I know this because, once we were big enough, that is all the clothes we wore. Anything that was slightly damaged in Burberrys would be put into bags to be given to homeless charities around New York City. But when my dad got involved, my mother would drive into the city and pick him up because he would bring bags of homeless clothes home for my mother to go through. The damage was always minimal, so we got loads of good stuff out of it at the expense of the needy.

Burberrys rebranded in 1999 and dropped the 's'. You would be amazed, the number of sweaters I have to this day that still have a 'Burberrys' tag on them. The stuff lasts forever – as does the guilt that some homeless guy froze in a New York winter so I could look preppy and rich when I was a youngster.

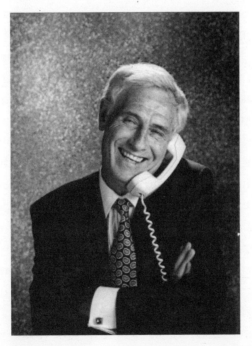

It looks like he is working but he is probably on the phone to my mother, telling her what time to collect him from the subway or the bus. We never liked it when he got the bus, because way too often he would wake up too late and miss his stop.

I am not sure exactly what my dad did in his job. It was a pretty big operation. In the early days there were five floors of shopping and quite a lot of staff, as well as a huge shipping and stock staff in the basement. My dad's skill was to make everyone feel important – from the basement guy to the department manager. I assume he had to deal with staffing and stuff like that, but I would say he had a lot of help with any of the logistical stuff, which was not really his strong point. Customer and staff relations were his forte, and he charmed the great and the good of Manhattan and all who came to visit.

When I say my dad was a showman I do not mean that he was loud or liked to tell jokes and attract loads of attention. I mean he was constantly aware of his image, both physically and in what people thought of him. The best example of this is the fact that he wore bronzer every day he went to work. As a boy I was clueless as to what he was doing every morning when he would put this tiny dot into his hand. Even the amount he squeezed out of the bottle was done with precision. This dot would then be rubbed into his hands to turn them a strange brown-orange colour, and then he would rub it into his face, making sure that he stretched this tiny dot into an even colour all the way down his neck. He would then wash his hands in almost the same way every morning after the application. I am sure if we had filmed his hand-washing, you would find it hard to spot any variation in time or pattern. He was obsessed with his image going to work and never deviated from this routine.

I asked him about it when I got older and he said unashamedly that a bit of bronzer made him look better on the floor at Burberrys. He was right too. The slight tan brought out his grey hair and strong features.

My dad spent a hell of a lot of time in the bathroom.

Much more than my mother or any of us. His time in the bathroom was ritualistic, but he had to perform his ritual amidst the traffic of everyone else popping in and out. We had only one bathroom, so you were not allowed to lock the door because if you were in the shower with the door locked, that meant that someone else would not be able to use the toilet. So in our house you just went ahead and used the toilet while the other person was in the shower. But you had to warn someone if you were using the sink because it affected the temperature of the water in the shower. Of course, it was funnier when you didn't warn them.

My dad would get in the shower first because he had so much stuff to do afterwards, and then we would use the bathroom while he was shaving, bronzing, brushing his teeth and combing his hair. He combed his hair in such a specific way and he used the same broken hairbrush for his entire career. It always went back into his mirror cabinet and no one else was allowed to use it. It was not a special hairbrush either. It was a cheap plastic one with the handle broken off, but it was his and it was always there in the same spot.

We pissed while he did it, and we showered while he did it. You did not even need to ask, but the minute you turned off the water in the shower, he would pass a towel over the top of the rail to you. It was almost as if he was not even thinking; the movements were almost robotic. You dried yourself off in the shower to stop water getting on the floor.

Then finally, when everyone was done, the cry would come down the stairs: 'Is everybody finished with the bathroom?' My dad needed to have everybody done because then he could lock the door. My father could not look after his business in the morning, knowing someone might use the toilet after him. He was very paranoid about the smell and all that went with it. Of all the things we joked about, the bathroom was a sacred place. He was very private about that. He was like clockwork too: he had set his digestive system to kick in once Aidan was done with the shower.

And to our horror, after it was over he would light a match and throw it in the toilet, the belief being that it got rid of smells. Personally, I always found that just made it worse, or at least gave my dad's business a distinctive smell. Of all the odours you want to have specific, that is not one of them.

He had the performer's nerves every day going to work, and he would torment my mother if things were running late. He could not handle a variation in the schedule. He could not handle letting people down. It was other people's approval that was of utmost importance. He was miserable if there was a delay, and you could feel the anxiety building once there was a chance he would be on a subway train ten minutes later than normal. The later subway would get him there on time, but it still did not stop him panicking.

Looking back, I got a real insight into my dad through going to work with him. I worked in Burberrys during the summer and for most Christmas sales from 1992 right up until the end of the decade. At the start he struggled with the commute because I did not hit the marks at exactly the right time. I did not put the token into the slot as quickly as him or remember to buy tokens on the Manhattan side in the morning when we arrived so we would not have to wait in the rush-hour line going home later that day. But eventually I figured out the routine. It was the same with my brothers when they ended up working there.

I loved the way every morning outside 179th Street station my dad made the *New York Post* guy smile by calling him 'my friend' before he got on the F Train. I loved the way everybody in Burberrys would always tell me what a lovely man my father was and how good he was as a boss. I was there long enough to have an awareness of the genuine affection everyone, from the stock room right through to the executives, had for him. But I think most of all I loved the performance in Burberrys myself. I loved the fact that because I could do my dad's accent perfectly I could entertain all the staff by mimicking his actions and words. I loved it when some of the higher-level executives asked me to 'do' my dad. I would really love it when he was there to see me in action and he enjoyed the way everyone was laughing. I did not take him off in an insulting way, and he never took it as an insult. I didn't realize it at the time, but really I was just a cliché: I loved going to work with my dad. (On top of that, for a teenager, I was a pretty good salesman of conservative male clothing. I banged out a load of bullshit to convince people they needed to spend $1,200 on a raincoat.) It was not just our family that worked with my dad in Burberrys. There must be at least twenty guys from our area who worked for my dad at some stage. Some of them still work there today.

Dad's obsession was 'making the day'. I assume making the day meant meeting the sales target for that day. I think the target was based on the previous year's sales for the corresponding day, but it may have been based on estimates. In the early years he always seemed to make the day. Most days, our welcome home to him would be: 'Did you make the day, Dad?'

In the early '90s my father's position came under threat. A number of people who wanted his job or in order to make space for their own advancement began to collude in having him removed from Burberrys. One of the pieces of ammunition used against him was that my father was unable to keep up with the modernization of systems when things had become more computerized. He went through a period of intense stress around this time and eventually he gave in to the pressure and took a demotion and went to manage the store at the Americana Mall in Manhasset, Long Island.

My father was very demoralized by this. Worse, after a year or two he ended up back in the New York store, but only to manage the men's department. Now he was working under the people he had once managed. I knew the people involved who plotted against him, but I was not experienced enough to understand how people could be that conniving. I used to obsess about one day making enough money so I could buy Burberrys and destroy one particular man's life.

For years I wondered why my dad did not tell those assholes to go fuck themselves and get himself a new job. But he had three boys, all needing to go to college, and all that goes with that. He took that shit and kept his head. I really felt bad for him at that time, while at the same time wishing he was more powerful and had not had to go through something like that.

In 1997 the top management team in Burberrys changed, and those executives who had conspired against my dad all got the sack. He was given a new position as head of customer relations. He really enjoyed those final years in Burberrys with less responsibility. He was adored by the new president, with whom he struck up a very strong friendship.

I was and remain very grateful to the management team that brought my dad back into the fold. What happened to him really affected his confidence, so it was a real triumph to know that he had been the victim of a heave. The fact that the new people saw him as indispensable meant so much to him. They called him Mr Burberry, and it was a huge part of his identity. He tried to retire and they would not let him. They accommodated him in every way, and for the last year or two they basically told him that all he had to do was come in and hang around and make people who were not happy feel better.

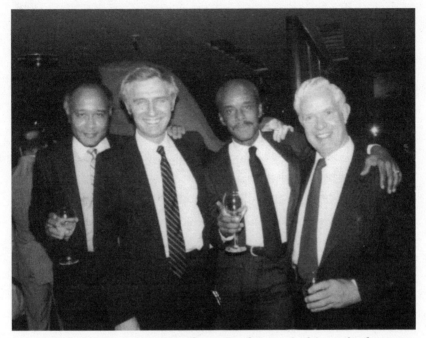

My dad with colleagues from Burberrys in his early days working there.

Finally he put his foot down and retired. My mother had a little bit to do with that. She was the one who had to take him to the subway every morning and pick him up every night, and she could not handle another winter of worrying about him walking in the snow. He had already had to have an angioplasty and was slowing down quite a bit. She couldn't handle the stress of him getting ready for his daily performance either. As he got older he got very set in his ways and would get extremely agitated if they left the house even a minute late. He did not want to let down his audience at work.

While I think retirement is overrated, I think in the end

my dad was happy to call it a day. He had worked Saturdays since 1977. He worked really hard too. All my life he told me that I should never get into retail, but I know that deep down he loved his job. I still see messages on my Facebook page from people who remember him in those final years when Irish people had more euros than they knew what to do with and would go in to get some Burberry to bring home. They would meet my dad, and the first thing he would ask them was if they had ever heard of me. He loved that. He loved telling me about it, too. He worried about my career, and I guess it temporarily put his mind at ease that I might just be doing all right.

Burberry organized buses throughout the day and evening to bring people to my father's wake. When all those Burberrys staff members and the company president turned up, it really got me. They were his fans and saw him as the soul of the store. It was such a lovely thing. He would have been delighted that they did that for him. He would have thought it was worth all the bronzer he put on to look good for them all those years.

One of the guys from the neighbourhood who got into Burberrys through my dad and who still works there says that people still come in asking for him. Some people come in looking for the Irish man, and some people come in looking for the English man. Even strangers could not figure out exactly who my dad was. But they always say charming.

Though he loved the job – once he was 'on', he loved the daily performance and having an audience – fairly early in my adult life I realized that my father always felt that his performance at Burberrys was something he had settled for, the price he paid for the stability he felt his family needed. After coming from the exciting London life of his twenties, the semi-suburban life we had in Flushing was a strange compromise for my father. He ended up in a working-class neighbourhood, far removed from the elegance he had known in his cosmopolitan past. It was a life of working Saturdays and inventory nights. I used to hate it when my mother would say, 'Your dad will be home late tonight, it's inventory night.' I knew that would mean my dad would be pissed off when he got home. He would eat his dinner in silence on his own, chewing his massive bites with venom.

I know that sometimes he regretted his decision and I could hear the discontent in his voice when he would tell me about the things he could have done. These regrets were not always about acting either. He told stories about owning a beauty salon in London with a former girlfriend, Valerie, at one stage, and also about having had the opportunity to buy a pub on the East side of Manhattan after he had married my mother. He always brought these things up when he got on a roll about missed opportunities. This was a common conversation all throughout my dad's life. Sometimes there was the arrogance of an insecure man trying to prove that he had once done or could have done amazing things. Other times there was just the tone of regret. It was always what could have been. The past seemed to bring the opposite of satisfaction for my father.

But my father had a ceiling in his mind and he believed that there was only so far he could go. There was an alarming number of things my dad felt he should have done. These thoughts were motivated by a creeping belief that he should not be here on 188th Street, licking ass for a living in Burberrys in a job in which he knew he could go no further because he had no real education. That ate away at him. The truth is that as I got older I realized that he saw a lot of his career as a sacrifice made for us. I must be honest and say that way too often he seemed unsure if the sacrifice was worth it.

When I was in my teens my father could see that I enjoyed working at Burberrys. He would turn to me and say, 'Just promise me you will never get into retail.' He probably worried less about me being an alcoholic than that.

13

My father talked a lot about the 'nearly James Bond' life in London, and he told us whimsical stories when we were growing up about playing hurling in cow shit in Midleton; but it was only after I stopped drinking at nineteen that he told me the truth about his upbringing. The first time he told me the story of his childhood we were out in the Hamptons. It was the summer of 1996 and I had been sober for a year, and that had brought us closer. I think it was just the two of us; my mother had gone back into Queens with the other two lads, most likely for something sports related, and me and my dad were just chilling out there together. We were sitting at the table and he began to tell me all these things about what really happened to him as a child.

Up to this point my understanding had been that he preferred Ireland to England as a boy and that his father was unable to be a parent as result of his wounds in World War II. This was the version he had decided was palatable for his young sons.

He told me it was around the time of the war that my father began to notice strange mood swings in his mother. Suddenly, without any explanation, he would get vicious smacks across the face, which came as a tremendous shock to him. Until this time, his mother had been a fun-loving, caring mother who spent a lot of time singing. His father, my grandfather, blamed this turn of events on the war. He was wounded at Dunkirk and had spent a long time recovering in a hospital in Folkestone in Kent, after which he was returned to light duties. As a result of his long absence it seems he was not aware of the full extent of the violence that was occurring in their home. I guess he thought she was under pressure, being effectively a single parent, and he must have lived in hope that she would somehow learn to cope better.

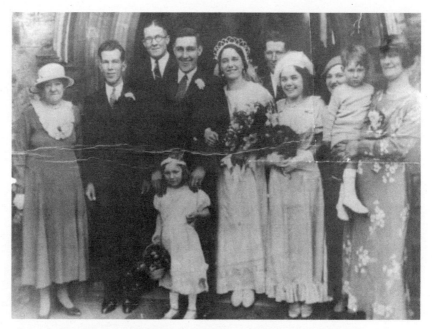

My dad's parents' wedding day. Stanley was the younger of the two and was still in his teens when he got married.

Despite the tragedy of my grandfather's wounds, for a number of years the war would bring a respite for my father from his mother's savagery. Churchill called for children who had relations in safer parts of the UK and Ireland to be sent there until the war was over, and my father was sent to his maternal grandparents in Midleton. Even before he left for Ireland, my father remembered a female neighbour in Bexhill telling his mother she would never be welcome in her house again if she did not stop beating her children.

So, on leave from light duty, my grandfather and grandmother brought my father and his sister Joan to Ireland on board the *Innisfallen*. After a few days, they left, leaving the children in the care of their uncles and my father's grandparents.

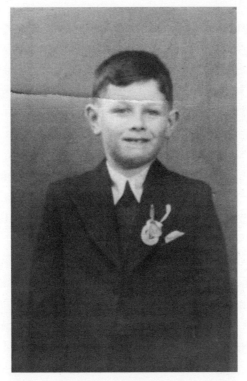

My dad's first communion portrait.

I always wondered why a man with an English accent would be so connected to Ireland. I always wondered why he held on to an almost mystical version of Ireland in his mind. But once I got a deeper understanding of his past, I could see that Ireland offered a respite from the chaos of his life back in England. Not only that, but his uncles and his grandmother absolutely adored him. I learned that later on, when I visited the house in Midleton. They spoke about him with deep affection and told wistful stories about his time there. Sadly, Ireland would always be the only place where my father experienced the love and safety a child should know. Though he never finished it, when he retired from Burberrys my father made an attempt at writing a memoir. It is full of warmth about his time in Midleton.

As a boy in Ireland I had a full working day with many chores to perform and going to school was not a top priority. Every day I would be woken up by my grandmother at 6 a.m. The house had no running water, so I would make three or four trips to the water pump up the lane and fill the white enamel buckets with water from the tap and drag it back to the house. My next chore was to scour the barn and the outhouses and collect the eggs where the chickens and geese had laid. I would then go into the forge and pump the bellows for my Uncle Willie as he shod the horses. Then I'd take the pony and cart, drive it to the poor house and pick up the offal, bring it back to feed the pigs. I would round up the cattle and bring them back for milking that evening. Milking the cows with my uncles was great fun. As they squeezed the milk into the buckets, they would play tunes and sing songs to the cows. They always squirted the milk in my face when I least expected it. My uncles William and Dick were always singing and making harmonies of Irish folk songs. There was always great laughter with me because my enemy around the farm was the gander and he was always trying to take a bite out of the arse of my pants. They would fall about with laughter when the gander tried to catch me.

A lot of men in the town were unemployed and they would stand on street corners wasting the day away. I recall one year that was a very tough year financially. The family had decided to grow barley and it was one of the worst summers, with belting rain every day, and the rain had flattened the barley and they managed to salvage just a few sacks. When they took the barley to the mills, they got only a few pounds for the entire crop. Many days I would have one potato in a saucer mashed in milk for dinner. I was always hungry. My grandmother would say, 'Times were hard,' but there was always laughter at the worst of times.

There was a great celebration when my Aunt Esther's third child was born. His name was Billy, and he survived because my Aunt Esther had gotten a council house on the land that my uncles had sold to the County Council to pay off some of my grandfather's debts. My Aunt Esther was overjoyed: there was no dampness, she had hot and cold running water, with a toilet and a bathtub. My grandmother considered it a tremendous luxury.

As an adult, married with three sons, it would break my heart to see my boys leave so much food on their plates. I would look at them and remember how hungry I always was at their ages.

The contrast with then and when that love and safety were violated is so strong when you read what happened when his mother came to visit Ireland to take the children back to England:

My mother came to Midleton to take my sister back to England, but I stayed another couple of years as my grandmother was very upset that I would have to leave. While my mother was staying for a few days, I ran out of the house and leaped in the air as if I was catching a ball and hit my head on the door jamb. My mother told me to go up into my room because I was punished. All those years in Ireland no one ever hit me, but my mother came into the room and gave me an unmerciful beating with a blackthorn stick and all hell broke loose in the house. My grandmother desperately tried to stop my mother, but she was a like a madman with superhuman strength. For the first time in my life I was absolutely terrified of my mother. My uncles came in and dragged my mother away from me and I was black and blue all over my body. My uncles said it was 'the ole fella [their father] all over again'. My mother left with my sister and peace and serenity came back into my life and I loved my wild, free childhood. My uncles would take me to Ballycotton and let me go where I wanted while they went to the pub. I always went up to the fields above the cliffs looking for wild mushrooms. I would whistle to myself and look out at the lighthouse without a care in the world.

The day inevitably came when my grandfather came to take my father home. His uncles did not want him to go, as he had become part of the family. My father definitely did not want to go as he feared the worst. He tried to hide in the woods under leaves, hoping the boat would leave without him, but his buddy Mickey Lee knew where he was and they found his hiding place. He had no choice but to go.

Things could not have got worse for my father. Sometimes I still find it hard to believe that some of those things happened to him. He returned to England with hardly any education, as his uncles never made him go to school. As a result, when he returned to Bexhill-on-Sea he was ridiculed in the school, unable to read and now with an Irish accent. Then he was sexually abused by a priest who taught in the Catholic primary school there:

My mother had her mind set on me becoming a priest and every day she would say to me, 'Many are called but few are chosen.' When Father Honan came into the classrooms looking for altar boys I was ecstatic that he had chosen me and my mother was over the moon with happiness as my mother went to Mass every morning and was a devout Catholic. After I became an altar boy, Father Honan took me down into the crypt and explained that I had to join his secret society. He took me into an old confessional box and asked me to drop my trousers and made the sign of the cross on my buttocks. I was to tell no one. As time progressed Father Honan would take me into his private room where he had grapes, which I had never tasted. He would give me grapes, take down my trousers and masturbate all over the cheeks of my buttocks. He made me hold his penis and other grotesque indecencies. When he was finished he would remind me that I was a member of the secret society and I could not tell anyone.

I knew nothing about the 'birds and the bees', but every time I left his private room I would have a sinking feeling; the only way to describe it was it was thick and heavy. Eventually one of the other altar boys told his parents what Father Honan was doing to him. His parents came to my father and my father asked me if he had done anything to me. I denied it at first, out of fear of my mother because she would never believe that a priest could do such a thing. My father kept on asking me to tell the truth and eventually I did tell him the truth about Father Honan and everything he did to me. The parents of the other altar boys were extremely angry and the parish sent Father Honan away. My mother stayed in complete denial.

As time went on, if anything went wrong, his mother

would give him terrible beatings and he developed a fear of grown-up men because of what had happened with the priest. In school he was distant and vacant and worried constantly about what would go on when he got home. His teachers could not understand why he could not learn, but he was too scared to tell them about the terrible violence that was being inflicted on him. His troubles in school only increased the excuses she had in order to beat him.

> When she learned that I was backward in school and had not caught up with the other kids sufficiently every day I would take a beating and be locked into the coal hole which was pitch black and in order to take away the fear of the darkness I would compose tunes by whistling until I was let out.
>
> My sister did not get the beatings that I received but she was very much affected by it because she would crouch into a corner and cry uncontrollably because she loved me so much and she could not bear to see me getting hit all the time. When she wouldn't stop crying for me my mother would grab her by the pigtails and drag her around the floor until she stopped crying.

The most disorientating thing was that as quickly as the violence came on, after half an hour his mother would hold him and cuddle him and tell him how much she loved him. When she would let him out of the coal hole, she would be all warm and friendly and joke with him that he looked like a chimney sweep. As the years went on and his mother's violence escalated, my father just tried to manage things.

> Over the years I learned never to enter the house without standing by the door and listening for her footsteps. If

her footsteps were heavy I knew that the violence would happen as soon as I entered the house, so I would go away and stay in the fields imitating the birds with my whistling and wait until darkness and come back to the house and stand outside and listen for the softer footsteps, then I would go in because I knew she would be happy and joke around. I stayed out of the house as much as I could and I joined the athletic club and in the club I joined the gymnastic team, the boxing team and I spent hours and hours playing soccer. Anything to stay away from her.

Unfortunately the beatings intensified and she progressed into beating me with a solid brass triangular stair rod. The rod had very sharp edges and I would try to protect myself with my elbows. The stair rod was the most painful beating of all. Sometimes my father would come home from work where he had a job off the books for a building company and try to protect me, but the more he tried to protect me, the worse my mother got. In her rage there were times when she would grab a saucepan full of boiling water and throw it at him. He would tell me to run and I would run out of the house and go back up into the fields and listen to the birds and imitate them with my whistling.

My father was a very simple man and just had no idea how to control her. In her rages she had superhuman strength and she was impossible to reason with, just completely out of control. I often wondered why my father didn't try to stop her more but then I would think that I was the reason why she was like she was. It was my fault that she went into these rages.

There was no respite. He suffered the indignity of failing all his entrance exams for secondary school and ended up in

97

the class for children with learning disabilities, and even in that class he was at the bottom. The only positive thing in his life was that he excelled in all the sports he played. This was partly down to the talent he was born with and partly down to his dedication to training, motivated by his desire to do anything to stay away from the house. At the age of eleven he won the 440-yard and 880-yard races in the school championships and he played for the South of England against the North of England; he was a centre forward and his goal-scoring prowess kept him in good graces with the schoolmasters, which made up for his total inability to progress academically.

And then the day came when he discovered his secret was not so secret after all. He had come home from school and, as he had always done, he listened for the sound of her footsteps.

The footsteps were quiet, but I had miscalculated. She had no shoes on. I walked in and sat down in the kitchen and she flew into one of her rages, went to the drawer and took out a carving knife. She started to slash me with the carving knife, I raised my arms to protect my face, the blood was all over my body and at that moment the front door flew open and two cruelty inspectors, two policemen and a nurse stormed into the house. Unknown to us the neighbours had made complaints and the inspectors and police were watching the house.

I remember the nurse wiping me down and bandaging my knife cuts. My mother was sitting in a chair, chain-smoking, just watching everything that was going on. My father walked in on all this. The cruelty inspectors asked me how the cuts happened and I told them that they happened while I was crawling through some barbed wire. My father realized that something had to be done, and whatever he said to the cruelty inspector, it ended up in my mother being immediately arrested.

My grandmother was refused bail and was held on remand in Holloway Prison until trial. My father was ordered to be taken to Dr Barnardo's Home for boys while a suitable foster home was found. My father watched as his mother was escorted to prison.

> I stood outside the courthouse waiting to be taken to Dr Barnardo's and I watched my mother being brought out handcuffed and put in the Black Maria with prison bars on the windows. She had her face to the windows holding onto the bars and as she was being driven away tears were streaming down her eyes and she mimed the words to me, 'I love you.' It was the worst feeling I ever had in my entire life.

Three weeks later she pleaded guilty to charges of child cruelty and was sentenced to two years' probation; she was committed to a mental hospital. Probation was on the condition that she go for treatment.

Local newspaper articles told the story of the years of abuse my father had had to endure. It was an awful thing to have everyone in Bexhill knowing what had happened. Of course the tragedy of it all is that my grandmother's illness would now be treatable. The shame was too much for my grandfather to handle and he took off for London and stayed away for over a year.

For my grandmother it was worse. She was sent to Hellingly Mental Asylum and there she was diagnosed with what my aunt called 'epilepsy of the brain' – paranoid schizophrenia. My father may have been the victim of her horrific abuse, but she was the victim of the way they treated people as violent as her in the mental health system of the 1950s. They decided to give her a lobotomy. When my father told me the story I thought it was really weird that my grandmother had had a lobotomy. Up until then, all I knew about lobotomies was that it was the thing that made McMurphy completely dumb and docile at the end of *One Flew Over The Cuckoo's Nest*.

*

TALK

...lanist, and during the war ran ... concert party for the troops ... Essex. With her husband, ...ho has always been interested ... the stage, she has helped to ...roduce plays presented by the ...ttenham Players at Banstead, ...urrey.

...arrow Escapes

Volunteering for the Merchant ...avy when war broke out in ...39, Mr. MacKenzie narrowly ...caped death on two occasions. ...e was serving as radio officer ...oard one of five ships ...tempting to reach besieged ...alta in 1941. It was an ...merican vessel, disguised as ...alian, but it was sunk by ...alian aircraft, together with ...e other four ships. A period of captivity followed ... Sfax, Southern Tunisia, but ...e landing of American forces ... Casablanca, in the west, was ...e prelude to Mr. MacKenzie's ...turn home. It was not for long, however, ... 1943 saw him back in the ...erchant Navy. As fate would ...ve it, the ship in which he ...as serving was sunk by a ...bmarine almost in the same ...sition as the boat he had been ...oard two years previously, ...d the injuries he then ...ceived put an end to his sea...ng service.

...issed the Point

In his letter to the "Obser-...r" last week, Councillor A. S. Stevens said that the onus ...s surely upon those members

MOTHER ADMITS WOUNDING SON

Remanded in Custody for Medical Report

WHEN Anne Bishop (40), of 65, Belle-hill, appeared on remand at Bexhill Magistrates' Court yesterday (Friday), charged with maliciously wounding her 15-year-old son, Michael Stanley Bishop, on August 16, she pleaded guilty. She also pleaded guilty to a further charge of wilfully assaulting and ill-treating the boy in a manner likely to cause unnecessary suffering and injury to his health, between March 1 and August 16.

ATTACKED WITH KNIFE

Mr. Norman White, prosecuting, said the case was one of unwarrantable violence and ill-treatment of the son over the past six months. Bishop had attacked the boy with her fists, a broom, poker, stair rod, and, finally, a knife. Her husband attributed the attacks to some sort of brain storm, and she had become worse since having an operation in March. In other ways she appeared to be a good mother to the children. The final attack was on August 16, when Bishop attacked her son with the flat of a knife, inflicting two cuts, one 3½in. long and the other 7½in. The following Sunday there was an attack with a clothes' horse, and the boy had left home. Accused had at first denied attacking her boy.

OUTBURSTS OF TEMPER

LETTERS

Hoteliers' Shortened

Sir,—In view of the sh... time available I request the ... of your columns to express ... Hotels Association's disquiet ... from the established practice exercising the option when the orchestra continues its ... formances until the end ... September. Bearing in mind the perso... knowledge of our members a... the requirements of the aver... visitor, the Council's decision regarded as a retrograde a... and one that will do a gr... deal of harm to the good re... tation built up for Bexhill ... ing the past few years. Co... cillors are asked to consider following points: 1. The presence and pleas... of an orchestra is a vital fac... when prospective visitors ... making up their minds whet... or not to come to Bexhill. 2. The sudden curtailmen... the orchestra's season will ... stitute in effect a misrepresen... tion to the large numbers ... visitors who come for the la... half of September and who h... been accustomed to the en... ment of the orchestra. S... treatment will undoubt... cause disappointment, if ... annoyance, and will result ... the killing of the habit of ... annual visit to Bexhill. 3. The late start and al... period of music is a great ... terrent as regards tempor... and permanent residence

My father claimed it was in the paper, so I found this in the *Bexhill Observer* from 30 August 1952.

That is more or less what my father told me when he first shared the story of his childhood with me. For some reason I had it in my head that the knife attack happened when he was about twelve, but checking things out for this book I've discovered he was fifteen. Not only do the records confirm everything he told me, but my Aunt Joan remembers it being just as bad as he said. She has very distinct memories of the day the police came to the house and arrested her mother. Hearing her talk about it was the first time I had heard the story of that day from another angle. It hit me hard because it confirmed that there was no dramatization in my dad's version of the tale. She also recalls the trauma of the whole story coming out in public after the court case. She recalls the embarrassment of walking into her art class in school and one of the girls in the class screaming out that she was the girl from the story in the paper.

My father ended up with a family called the Wallaces, and Joan went to the Mitchells. She remembers horrible trips to the mental hospital in Hellingly and walking by all the padded cells to go and visit her mother with her father when he came back on the scene. My father also had vivid memories of those visits:

> I became very depressed when I finally walked in to the ward that my mother was in. The only way they knew how to calm the patients down was with shock treatment and it seemed they gave my mother very high dosages. All the women in that ward had straight hair and they would shuffle around. They thought that the war was still on and the curtains must be drawn otherwise the Germans would see the light coming through the curtains and they would be bombed. That was the first time my mother said to me that I was a detective trying to poison her tea and she would continue to say that for years and years and years.

My grandfather drank his way through much of this whole ordeal. He disappeared for a while, but when he returned and my grandmother got out of hospital for a spell, there was an attempt to return to normal life. However, she quickly returned to the way she had been – one night she was found in the nearby village of Sidley, walking around in her nightdress, and she was returned to Hellingly – and the children went back into foster care. She spent seven years in Hellingly altogether. My grandparents lived together again after she got out of hospital and they stayed together until he died in 1976. She was in and out of institutions the entire time. Despite that, for much of that time they visited Ireland every September, and most of my relations were kept in the dark about the severity of what had happened.

Aunt Joan realized quite late in life that in fact her dad had been an alcoholic. When I reread my dad's writings, following our conversation, for the first time I could see that he was aware of it too:

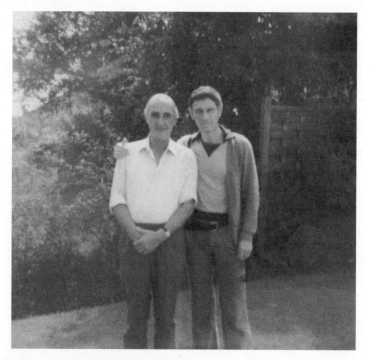

My dad and his dad in Bexhill in 1975, when I was on the way.

I realize now that my father was a very weak man and just could not help us, he didn't know what to do so he always just ran from us and from trouble. He never faced what was going on, he just ran from it all. I did love my father but there was always that barrier in my mind of why he let what happened to me happen. I always thought that perhaps it was because he lost his father at Battle of the Somme in the First World War. I always just tried to make that as an excuse for his weakness.

I have since asked my mother, and she remembered that when my grandfather visited New York in 1976, a short time before he died, most days he went to the pub for a few drinks on his own. I get the impression he was a very gentle and lovable drunk, though, and never really fell out with anyone through drunkenness. My mother remembered that he made friends very quickly during his time in Queens. I know that it meant a lot to my dad that his father got to see me before he died. I don't think they ever had any real resolution though.

14

There were a few parts of my dad's story from his memoir that I found hard to make sense of. He wrote about a time when he was a bit lost and living in London with criminals and alcoholics. But this didn't seem to fit his timeline; he seemed to be suggesting that he ran away from the foster home at the age of sixteen and went to London. From Joan I now know that this period in his life was much later, actually in his twenties, after he got out of the hospital after hurting his back.

Joan lost contact with my father after he got out of the hospital, and it took her a while to track him down to London. When she went to see him, he was quite down and out, heavily alcoholic and living in squalid conditions. This was before he had begun modelling. She credits a man called Roy for saving him because he got him into modelling. From what she saw in London when she visited him, she is convinced that without Roy's intervention my dad would have been lost forever.

The stories my dad wrote about his early years in London are very confusing. It is my belief that his account here is a combination of how he joined the army and his time in London. I don't think he was in London between the ages of sixteen and eighteen, because that was when he joined the Sussex Regiment, his local regiment, to do his National Service:

After I would pay my foster parents for my keep,
I managed to save a few pounds for myself. One

afternoon I finished work earlier than usual and walked in on a conversation that my foster mother was having with a group of her friends. They never heard me coming because I walked very silently, a habit I got into so that my mother would not hear me coming home. She was telling them that I was eating too much peanut butter from the jar and that her husband Bert was extremely cross with me. I crept up to my room, packed a small suitcase, shimmied down the drainpipe and boarded a train to London and found my way to the steps of the Chelsea Town Hall in the King's Road. For two nights I slept on the park benches in the King's Road. At night there was always a bunch of teenagers sitting on the steps, and from there they would go into the snooker halls. I followed them in one night and struck up a conversation with a boy called Jimmy Keane, whose mother was Irish. He knew I had nowhere to stay so he took me home to his mother and I stayed a few nights. She was very kind to me. I walked around the building sites in Kensington where a lot of demolition was going on. I lied about my age and got a job wheeling barrowloads of rubble into lorries. Finally, I found a room in Putney, sharing it with a fellow two years older than me called Sean Brady, who was also a labourer on the construction sites and was from Dublin.

Brady was a very heavy drinker and by Monday morning he would be flat broke. He would get a sub from the foreman till his next paycheck on Thursday. I would go off to the pubs with Brady and I used to drink, hoping that I could hold my beer like Brady could. We always went to pubs where there was a piano player and a singer. One night I jumped up to the microphone.

In those days there was a very popular artist by the name of Ronnie Ronalde who used to whistle 'In a Monastery Garden'. The piano player would ripple through the chords, and Ronalde would imitate bird sounds. I used to do a very good impersonation of him. The piano players loved me because they could ripple up and down the keyboards while I was imitating bird sounds. I would drink for free. Brady loved going to the pubs with me because he would be included in the free drinks. Unfortunately Brady started to get homesick for Dublin, going from one extreme to the other to save every penny – he wouldn't even buy new socks, or a bar of soap, and his feet used to stink. One day he upped and left, owing the landlady a week's rent, and he stuck me with having to pay it. Life became very lonely for me after that.

The demolition job I had no longer needed labourers and my money started to run out. I would go to Victoria Station and stand there all night, feeling very lonely and hoping I would see a face that I recognized. I would make my way up to Piccadilly and hang out in the snooker halls and talk to broken-down boxers. They were the only friends I had. A boxer called Tommy Burke told me the worst thing I could do was to go through life feeling sorry for myself and that my eyes were oozing self-pity. After he told me that I made up my mind that I would never feel sorry for myself again. He introduced me to a man who had a window-cleaning company and told him that I was looking for work and he gave me a job.

The owner of the window-cleaning company, Tommy the Scrum, rolled his own cigarettes very, very thin like a matchstick. He told me, 'That's how you roll 'em in prison.' Everyone that worked for him had done time. He treated me like his own son and he protected me. I never forgot his kindness. This crowd were also heavy drinkers. It felt like winning a gold medal when they told me that for a young lad I could really hold my beer. On a Saturday we would finish cleaning windows at noon, and we would go to the pub and drink till three o'clock in the afternoon. On this particular day the thought of going back to my room and being alone again was too much. That afternoon I walked into an army recruiting centre and signed up to the British Army for twenty-two years.

When I told Tommy the Scrum that I had signed on to the British Army, he said it was an insane thing to do, 'But now that you have done it, you've made your bed and you will have to lie in it.'

What Tommy didn't realize was that I'd signed up out of loneliness and desperation. What also prompted me to do it was I had a belly full of beer at the time.

I knew that my dad had known some of London's criminals; it just never made sense to me until I read this. My father was very friendly with Terry 'Lucky Tel' Hogan, a notorious and very successful thief in London. Terry was the best friend of Bruce Reynolds, who mastermined the Great Train Robbery. It seems like my dad might have just been name-dropping, but I have seen a photograph of my parents with Terry Hogan and his second wife on holidays together in Hastings while my mother was pregnant with me. My mother remembers visiting his amazing house and she also remembers how good Terry's wife was to her when she was pregnant. She visited her all the time.

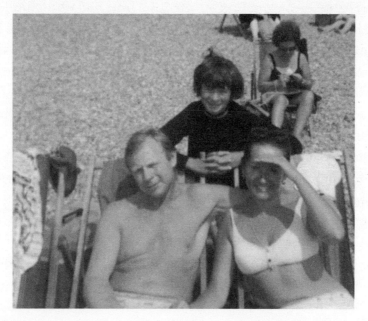

Terry Hogan, his second wife Roz and son Keith while on holiday with my parents in Hastings in 1975. Keith remained in contact with my father and stayed in our house in New York while I was in Ireland. Sadly, Terry committed suicide in 1995. Bruce Reynolds spoke at his funeral and Keith sent us a picture of his family with Bruce at the winning post at Aintree, where they spread his ashes.

My father knew all those characters from the London underworld. I just never understood how and why he met them. Now it makes sense that before he got into modelling, like many kids who went through what he did, he found himself in London in the shadier circles, working on building sites and hanging around pool halls. (He was very good at pool. Every time he hit a shot he would always say, 'Sign of a misspent youth!' I would say now it was a sign of a life story untold.)

I am not surprised though that the story about peanut

butter was the catalyst for him to remove himself from Bexhill. He was always talking about that moment.

One of the reasons my dad wanted to place himself in London when he was much younger was because he loved *Oliver Twist* and he loved London. I think he wanted to see himself as the young Oliver, fleeing tyranny to London. When my dad went to write his memoir he tried to fit the experiences of his life into narratives he was familiar with. Essentially he had no belief in his life being interesting enough without these embellishments and half-truths.

My father did not want people to know that he had only been in Ireland for four years during the war. He did not want people to know that his years of struggling in London did not take place until his mid-twenties. He did not want to admit that he had been back living with his parents in Bexhill after the army, but in fact that was the case. I don't know why it was the case, because it makes even the story of him breaking his back all the more tragic. Yet it may have been what saved him because it got him out of Bexhill.

Once my dad moved to London he would never return to live in Bexhill again either in reality or in his memory. It is understandable that he would eradicate as much of Bexhill from his story as he could. It was horrific. By the time he came to writing a memoir, he had forgotten the truth to a certain extent. He had a story in his mind that he told the world, and he nearly believed it himself.

PART TWO

. . . Like Son

I was the youngest of my friends on our block and I was the last one to start proper school, so they had all gone into first grade and beyond by the time I was in kindergarten. I have a vivid memory from this time. I can see the four-year-old me standing in the alleyway where we always played and it is still warm in the late September sun. It is so quiet and still. There is literally no one anywhere, which I see as eerie because I know the alley only as a place of noise and play. I have to squint, it is so bright. I can see the clothes hanging off the lines in rows, gently flapping in the midday sun and their shadows dancing on the asphalt.

I walk to the alley at the other side. I look down there, and again there is nothing to greet me but clothes and the barking of the Fullers' dog, which has smelled me from four houses away. I can hear the leaves in the breeze and it's the first time I am ever aware of them because I have never experienced such quiet. It is too quiet and all I can feel is a terrible loneliness and a longing for my friends to return. I go and stand on the corner of 189th Street to wait for the school bus to return to the corner, but it's hours away.

After a while I give up and I walk back towards my house. I don't know why, but I don't want to go in there. I feel a terrible anxiety and I am aware of it clearly. Something just doesn't feel right. I stand there and I listen to the trees and I hum to myself, but all the time I am thinking: what is wrong with me? My mother was inside watching the soap opera *All My Children*, yet I was more comfortable in this lonely isolation than in my home.

I can't help but notice that for much of my life I wished I was somewhere else. I can't say why I was already searching for something at that age. But this is not the beginning of a story about blame. It is a story about not being comfortable in the places where we should have been safe.

15

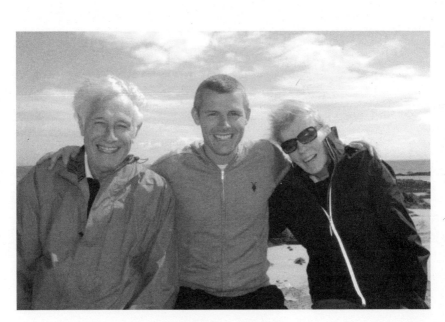

Connemara, 2008.

Becoming the parent of my parents was a real education. It was the first time that I really put someone else's welfare before my own. My mission in life was to make sure that my dad would be OK and that my mother had enough help to get through everything. I am a natural procrastinator, but very early on I realized that would have to change if I was going to help my dad. I knew I had to make awkward phone calls. I knew that I had to do some research to make sure my dad was getting the best care. I knew I had to cancel gigs I did not want to cancel. I knew that for the time being my life was no longer mine.

In real terms this was nothing like the sacrifice of parenting. For starters there were four of us helping each other out, and thankfully my dad was not helpless. He was still able to do things and did not need round-the-clock care. My mother was also very capable, and very soon after my dad got sick she pulled herself together and began to organize things in an almost obsessive-compulsive way.

It was still a real eye-opener for me to know that when the buck stops with you, the only option is to act. I had to force my dad to eat when he didn't want to and would snap at me. My dad could get very sharp at times when I would try to force him to have a few sips of the nutrition shakes we had for him. 'Ah, for fuck's sake; are we going to start with this bullshit again?' It was tough to have to fight with him over our desire to help him survive. I can't identify with his aversion to eating because I have never been in his situation, but I can tell you that for the first few weeks, when the weight was falling off him, at times he was violently opposed to eating.

My mother would be nearly crying downstairs, she was so worried about him not eating. She would ask me to try to persuade him to eat because she thought he would not want to let me down. That worked only twice, and then he realized that I was taking over my mother's role and that he would have to treat me with the same disdain. The doctors had told me it was essential that my dad ate, because he would need the strength to get through the chemo. They had told me that at that point in time not eating was actually the greatest threat to his survival.

We had some great battles back then and, to be honest, I liked the dynamic. When I say that, I mean I liked having to be strong enough to not give in to him. I would try and shame him by asking him if he wanted to die. I told him that it was no problem if that was what he wanted, but he would need to let us know so we could prepare.

'Just one more sip, please!' We all joked that we could play airplane if he thought it would help. It really is an incredible role change when you end up feeding your dad. It just makes you closer really. In the end my dad was very grateful, and finally he got his appetite back. He ended up putting on so much weight that his vanity took over and he began to worry that he did not look great. I think he worried about that more than about dying. Often he would stand in front of the mirror and grab his belly. 'Look at that gut. Look!' The first thing he told everyone who came over was that the oncologist said she liked her patients to be pudgy. He was probably thinking that everyone's first thought was, 'Wow, Mike has put on some weight!' Of course what they were thinking was, 'Wow, Mike is looking great for someone who is dying!' but you can see what my dad's priorities were; even when he was dying he was worried about his image.

When I was growing up, my mother used to love to say, 'One day you will understand.' That was her favourite expression. She did not say it to get out of having to explain something; it was always when we were challenging her as to why we could not do something or why we were in so much trouble for something. We were like professional footballers when it came to challenging our parents over some perceived injustice. We were up in the referee's face for every decision, and we could rarely see what we had done wrong. As with all referees, they made the odd mistake; but their decisions, whether correct or not, stood. Like most referees, their intentions were noble despite their imperfections.

The other thing my mother used to say and do when she was really stressed out was to look up to the heavens and exclaim, 'What am I am going to do with these children?', or, 'Please, God, give me the strength to deal with these children!' You could see the stress in her mouth as she said it. My mother used to store all her tension in her jaw. When I clench my teeth I think of my mother. It seemed that this was her expression most of the time. My mother's sisters were the same. It's an O'Hare trait. If I was joking around about making a movie about my brothers and my cousins swimming in calm water where no parents were around, and that calmness turning to terror when they showed up, we would have no problem calling it *Jaws*.

As I got older I knew the moment would come when I actually would understand what my mother meant. Life had given me enough insight to know that I was a hyperactive hothead who was hard to handle. Maturity and sobriety had made me a more peaceful guy and I had begun to understand a few things. But I assumed that the real moment of understanding would come when I had a child myself. I always thought that this is when the grandparents really get their revenge. This is when they get to watch you try to organize life with a crying baby in one room and a jealous toddler in the other. This is when they get to watch you try to break up a fight and make both children feel like they won. This is when they get to tell you how much better than you they were at all that stuff. This is how the cliché goes as far as I was concerned.

I see it with my brother's kids and my cousins' kids. The grandparents love making comments about things they would not let the kids do. They are very critical.

But the moment I figured out what my mother meant was when I became the parent of my parents and I knew that they had become dependent on us. My life flashed before my eyes and I could see my entire existence in a new light. I realized I had spent my life telling my parents to relax as much as I possibly could.

Found passed out, drunk, on the kitchen table in my own vomit on the eve of Mother's Day, 1990: 'Relax!'

Kicked out of school at fourteen years old: 'Relax!'

Drug problem at nineteen: 'Relax!'

Testicular cancer at twenty-four years old: 'Relax!'

I could not tell my mother to relax enough, truth be told. It was as if I thought I was the Dalai Lama.

Now I was feeding my father, cleaning my father, taking him to the doctor. Plus I was trying to keep my mother from imploding while also making her feel like she still mattered. My dad was like one child getting all the attention, and my mother was like the other, stomping her feet and thinking, 'What about me?' My mother has her own health issues, so I would offer to take her to the doctor and then for coffee, but she would say, 'No, we have to get back to your father.' Of course I was thinking, 'No, actually you need to look after yourself because Dad is just chilling and watching football and you are just stressing yourself out.' But of course I didn't say anything because, like a parent, I was trying to be especially patient.

My father would snap at my mother a lot during the day. He took much of his frustration out on her. My mother made a lot of pained noises and pulled a lot of pained faces and then, when you asked her what was going on, she would say that nothing was wrong. You could not get her to admit a thing. Instead, there would just be this tense atmosphere around the place. You just got the sense that, if she admitted a thing, she would just break down and cry. I wished that she would. It would have been the appropriate response.

'Mom, why don't you come to the movies?'

'No. Desmond. There . . . Is . . . Just . . . Too . . . Much . . . Stuff . . . I . . . Have . . . To . . . DO!'

She would emphasize each word, as if asking her to go to the movies was some sort of insult. There was nothing she really had to do other than sit still, which she was incapable of doing. So she would be making her noises and my dad would be refusing to drink water, despite the fact that on a few occasions we had to bring him to the hospital to get hydrated. Once or twice I found myself looking up to the heavens and thinking, 'What am I going to do with these children?'

Or my new personal favourite cry for help: 'MAYDAY! MAYDAY! Please talk us down.'

The day had come when I really understood. In fact, after a few weeks of my dad being sick, my mother turned to me and said, 'Desmond, you need to relax.'

You fucking relax! One day you will understand . . .

16

As I said, this is not a story about blame and I will spare you the details of how I ended up such an uncomfortable teenager, but something had been building up in me from a very young age. It managed to stay beneath the surface for years, but when the hormones of adolescence kicked in my emotional life exploded.

I have joked in my shows for years about how I ended up coming to live in Ireland at fourteen. The joke is that I got kicked out of school because I had a problem with alcohol and my mother came up with the ingenious idea of sending me to Ireland to go to boarding school. Of all the countries in the world . . . perhaps she saw potential in my alcoholism and wanted to make me the best alcoholic I could be. Ireland was the premiership, and if I was showing this much talent so young, I would need to be among the best if I wanted to progress. It was as if I was the Wayne Rooney of drinking.

It's not really true, though. Yes, I already had a drinking problem at the age of fourteen, but it was only one factor in my coming to Ireland and a small one in getting kicked out of school. The drinking was just a symptom of something deep within me that was very discontented.

The first problem was that I started drinking at twelve years old. I was the youngest of the gang of us who hung around together in the neighbourhood, and some of them were already sixteen during the summer of 1988. So when they started drinking, I started drinking. It was innocent enough for them — they were just teenagers having a few beers in the park – but I wasn't a teenager yet. The other problem was, I was the product of multi-generational alcoholism on both sides. I had 'the gene', as my mother would call it, and once I let that genie out of the lamp I didn't need three wishes because I had only one: MORE!

I can still recall how it felt that first night I got drunk. *I don't feel twelve. I feel like a man. My mind is empty and the questions ease. I can see the corner of 188th Street and 47th Avenue illuminated under the street light. I can see the trees. They look so beautiful and still. I want to stare at them for ages. I feel still, too. I have no anxiety. It is the greatest night of my life . . .*

In the summer of 1989 I began drinking a lot more. I had major blackouts and it was miraculous that I did not get caught by my parents. I wet the bed from total drunkenness for the first time and I remember telling my mother that I must have had a wet dream. I will always remember what she said because, despite the seriousness of the situation, it was really very funny. 'I don't know what kind of man you think you are, but wet dreams don't soak all the way through the mattress!' I thought I was busted for sure, but I guess she was not ready to admit what was really going on.

The real reason I wound up wanting to go to another country had a lot less to do with booze, however. I went to high school in the fall of 1989. Most of my friends had gone to another high school, so I did not know many people when I got to St Francis Prep. It was a high school with three thousand kids, and half of them were girls. All three thousand of us were dealing with more hormones than the Tour de France. I joined their ranks and for some reason I was not equipped to fit in.

Within a few months of being there I experienced two major instances of what people today would say was clearly bullying, but back then nobody used that term. First, this

Italian-American kid developed a serious crush on my girl-friend and started to make my life a misery. He knew all of the Howard Beach kids, the largest group in the school, and I knew hardly anyone. Suddenly, every day I was going to school afraid of these kids.

If that was not bad enough, my best friend who had gone to another school fell in with a new crowd. No sooner had I found a way to deal with the intimidation in school than my friend and his new gang turned on me. By Christmas I had lost all my confidence, my interest in school disappeared and I was failing loads of subjects. To add to the problems, as a result of the rejection of these groups I started hanging out with the neighbourhood kids every weekend. That meant drinking every weekend. My life became drinking, figuring out ways to lie to my parents about how school was going and hanging out with my girlfriend. The sense of exclusion was excruciating.

Since my very young days I had had the feeling that some-thing was not right with me. I could not put my finger on it, but it was with me so often. Now these feelings were veri-fied. There was something wrong with me and everyone else had figured it out. I would sit on the couch at night in our living room. We only used it when people were over so it was a very quiet room. I would sit there and pray for the phone to ring. I would wish that someone wanted to be with me. I could feel the emotion in my ankles and my fingertips, it was so strong. Sometimes it almost paralysed me. I wanted to fit in so bad.

On the eve of Mother's Day, 1990, my parents came back from a wedding very late to find me passed out, drunk, in my own puke on the kitchen table. This was more teenage drama than *Beverly Hills, 90210*.

I had been put on academic probation in school, and

a few months later the inevitable happened: St Francis Prep informed us that I had been expelled due to inadequate academic performance.

A few weeks later my parents found me blacked out, drunk, for the second time. I actually came home and pissed in the fireplace in our house in Westhampton. I have no recollection of it whatsoever.

It must have been tough on my dad because these were the things he used to do himself when he would black out. Initially he said nothing much at all. Then weeks later he got angry at me over nothing. I said, 'What the fuck is your problem?'

He got really angry and got right into my face, his chest nearly touching mine as he shouted, 'My problem is you coming home here drunk and wetting the bed and getting kicked out of school and thinking that you haven't done anything wrong!' He said many things that had been building up. I think he told me I was full of piss and wind as well. I know that it was pretty intense and was one of the only times I really thought my dad was going to kick my ass. I stood up to him as if I was ready to fight him, but I was actually freaked out by his anger.

My mother knew that I was an alcoholic. She had been around it her whole life and she could recognize 'the gene'. This time when they caught me, drunk, my mother told me quite calmly, 'Desmond, you don't know it yet, but you are an alcoholic and it is going to bring you so much pain.'

I remember giving her a smartass answer and saying, 'What do you want me to do, go to AA?'

I would like to think she said, 'One day you will understand!' But I know that at that point she had no time for my arrogance. She was not really angry that second time, she was just disappointed and upset because she knew that now she would have to deal with a third generation of alcoholism in her life. She had been surrounded by it from birth, and it was refusing to leave her alone. Looking back, I guess I was lucky that my mother was so good at letting me know when I was really young that I was screwed with the booze, so I never really had a chance to be in denial for too long.

I was in Queens in 1990; it was on the fringes of New York City. It was at the edge of a time when crime was rampant and crack was king. Though we lived in the semi-suburban quiet of eastern Flushing, the dysfunction of the city leaked into our safe, tree-lined world. Many people who were close to our family, including extended family members, had graduated from graffiti-writing, robbing cars and gang violence, to cocaine and crack addiction. People had no faith in the public school system which was now the only option open to me after being expelled. You could succeed there, but the cracks to fall through were wide. It was not a safe place for an impressionable young kid like me who was attracted to all the wrong things.

I can't really say why I was so uncomfortable in my skin at that time, but I knew I was on a bad road. I was desperate for attention and acceptance after the rejection of my friends. I don't really know if there was anything my parents could have done at the time. It was in this atmosphere of chaos and confusion that the idea of moving to Ireland came up.

On the day that Ireland beat Romania in the World Cup, I got the letter with the official word that I had been kicked out of school. I had to call my mother with the news and she broke down crying. But she stopped crying when I told her that Ireland was in a penalty shoot-out with Romania. I had to give her a play-by-play of the shoot-out, and when David O'Leary popped it in the back of the net, she was happy for a moment, and then she went back to crying.

'Desmond, what are we going to do with you?' This was a genuine *disasta*.

That summer, a cousin – Fiona Treanor, the daughter of my father's first cousin Marie – was visiting us on her way to Cape Cod to work for the summer on a J1 visa. Having been kicked out of school, I was in summer school and she was helping me with my homework. We were unsure where I was going to go to school after that, and Fiona suggested that maybe I could go to school in Ireland. I thought it was a great idea. I could not get out of New York fast enough. I was incredibly miserable and I thought anywhere would be better than there.

I told my parents and at first they just laughed. But then they turned to my godfather, Eamon Doran, for advice. His own kids had a very transatlantic existence and he thought it would be a great thing for me who had become so distracted. Because Eamon was a big fan of me going to Ireland, so was my dad. My father really trusted Eamon's opinion. It is understandable really that my dad would think that me going to Ireland was a good idea. It was the only time he was happy in his childhood so I am sure he thought I might find happiness there too.

For both my parents it seemed quite a prestigious thing to do. They both liked the idea that I was going to boarding school abroad. The perception of boarding school in the States was very elite. Due to the difference in the standard of living between Ireland and America in 1990, boarding school in Ireland seemed quite affordable. St Francis Prep was pretty expensive anyway. To them, it was a cheap way to offer a very prestigious solution to my problems in education.

Fiona's dad Tom came back with loads of information on St Peter's College in Wexford, where he himself had gone, and the final decision was made after I had a conversation on the phone with St Peter's principal, Fr Donal Collins. He asked me a few questions about myself and why I had been kicked out of school. He seemed happy with the conversation and he said he could see no reason why I should not be happy there. (As it turned out, he was aware of a few reasons why some kids might not be happy there, because he was sexually abusing them. He would later go to prison and was one of the three main priests featured in the Ferns Report into clerical abuse in the diocese.) It literally all took place over a six-week period, from the day it came up with Fiona to me leaving. Suddenly that was it; I was going to Ireland.

My mother told me recently that she said to my father before I went to Ireland that I was going to have to go through whatever journey I was going to have with booze. She had no idea what that journey would be, but she thought that I would be safer there. She had seen what our neighbourhood had done to the children of people she had known, and she thought that Ireland would be a place where I would get in less trouble. She truly thought that if I stayed in Queens I would end up either in jail or dead.

I knew nothing of my dad's past then. I had no idea that in much more dramatic circumstances he had ended up living away from his parents at exactly the same age as me.

17

Part of my wanting to tell this story is because I wanted to make sense of my dad's life. There were parts of his life he did not want us to know about for a long time. I eventually accepted that my father had a narrative about his past that he had come to accept. Still, it was a narrative with gaping holes in it. There were always holes because, even when my dad was there, he wasn't there. It's hard to locate those vivid memories of a man who is lost in his thoughts.

First thing in the morning, before his routine in the bathroom, my father would come downstairs to get a cup of coffee. He would often sit there, just staring out the window on to 188th Street. You could come down the stairs and pass him and he would pay no attention to you at all. There is nothing on 188th to absorb that much attention, so you knew he was in some other place. Sometimes he would be shaking his head and often he would start talking to himself. He would completely forget where he was.

When I think of how often we would find my dad pacing in car parks while we were shopping, his hands clasped behind his back or, smoking, lost in some other place, it seemed like he was only coming along for the ride. Once, on the way to the Hamptons, we all went into a 7/11 and he stayed outside to pace and smoke and think and talk to himself. While we were in there a woman came in and said to the cashier, 'There's a crazy man outside walking in the car park.' We realized she was talking about our dad. At times he was like a hitchhiker on our family's journey, a quiet presence who didn't like to get too involved.

He just didn't know how to do it. All our lives he would say to us, 'One of these days I am going to take you to Great Adventure' or 'One of these days I am going to take you bowling.' I guess it would have been on one of those days when he got a driver's licence. But the day never came.

I assumed those gaps in his story were filled with the things we didn't know about his past. But then I thought about the story of our relationship and there's a hole there too. I kind of noticed it by accident. When I say that, I mean that I am aware I spent my teenage years in Ireland away from my family, but I honestly didn't realize until I sat down to write this story how much of a gap it creates. I then noticed that, without it being intentional, I had jumped from the age of fourteen to my dad getting sick in the stage show, with no mention of what comes in between. I didn't even want to get into explaining all those years we spent apart. It was a story I was not comfortable telling. I guess, like my dad, I was worried about the judgements others would make.

Because of the hole in my story, I think that is why it was so important for me to spend so much time with my dad later on. I was the absent son. I needed to be present. Maybe he thought he was the absent father.

I pretend the gap in my story is not there and try to talk about things in a way that no one will notice. It is one manifestation of the distance that grew in our family. Many kids are sent to boarding school and perhaps they don't always feel so separate, but there is a strange thing about going to boarding school in another country that makes you feel apart. There are so many experiences when no one is there.

I left New York as an unaccompanied minor on Aer Lingus flight 104 on the evening of 25 August 1990. I was fourteen years old and had never been outside the United States since arriving when I was less than one month old. I was going to an entirely new culture on my own with hardly a pubic hair to show for myself, to be met by cousins I had never met before. I thought I was much wiser than my fourteen years and I was not afraid.

Now, when I think about writing down stories about my father, I can feel that distance when I think of all those years when I never turned to my parents. They did their job in the way they thought was best. Nothing was ever dealt with calmly in our house. It was a dramatic situation, and they responded to it in a dramatic way. There was nothing about me at the time that suggested I would end up loving Ireland and staying. My mother always says that she thought I would only last a semester, and she really hadn't planned on me staying.

The strange thing is that they never even saw St Peter's. The first time they came to see me in Ireland was for my graduation from University College, Cork, in 1998 (which they should have been very proud of because it took me two extra years to get there). They did not really get involved in any of the big decisions in my life. I did not have to ask their permission to do things. I did not have to show them my homework. They weren't there to help me with my Leaving Cert. They were not there to help me choose a college. If I mentioned the letters CAO* they would not have known what those letters mean. They were not there when I got my results. They were not there to help me find a place to stay in Cork. They could not even visualize all those years of my life. They had very little context.

This is not something I am upset over, it is just a state-

---

* Central Applications Office – the Irish clearing organization for third-level education courses

ment of fact. They were not part of that story. And believe me, at the time I was not wishing for them to be around. I had plenty to be getting on with that I did not want my parents knowing about.

It is not so much about them not doing their job; it's more about all the moments when they were absent. It brings with it a loneliness; it brings with it memories of a premature independence that was joyous and sad in equal measure. I used to tell my cousins in Waterford with whom I stayed at the weekends that I would be staying with school friends the following weekend. I would have no idea who I would be staying with, though – I would just find out who had big plans the following weekend, and go and stay with them. I once had nowhere to stay and ended up sleeping in the gate lodge of the cemetery in Crosstown, County Wexford, because some of my school friends would often use it as a place to get drunk at weekends. I was going out with a girl then who lived around there, and I remember walking up and down the road to pass the time because I knew I could not call around to her until after eleven o'clock. Her mother had seen me strolling around and the girl told me afterwards that her mother was concerned that I had no one wondering where I was.

But nobody was wondering, because nobody knew where I was. I was pretending to be somewhere else. All I had to do was check in with my parents on a Saturday, which in those days I could do from a payphone. My mother would just call me back wherever I was. On the surface there was nothing to worry about. I had become a good student and was on the Student Council. There were never many bad reports going back to them.

For me it's all about the peanut butter. When I finally got a chance to read my father's abandoned memoir, of all the things that stood out for me it was the moment he writes about when he overheard his foster parents discussing the fact that my dad ate too much peanut butter. There is nothing worse than that feeling of being a burden. I had that feeling many times while I was in Ireland. I would never disrespect the people who looked after me. They took me in and welcomed me, but there are always times when you feel you are a burden in a place where you don't belong. My father never knew a safe place called home. He was forced into a place where peanut butter became an issue. I chose to leave home too and ended up feeling the same way. My father always talked about the peanut butter story after he revealed his past to us. For him that was the breaking point. After everything he'd been through he wasn't worth forgiving for eating peanut butter from a jar.

I wanted to run from Queens back then when I was fourteen. That's why I was so happy to come to Ireland. I was so discontented and I did not even know why. I don't have any regrets about those years of independence, though, as I feel they turned me into the person I am. It definitely accelerated my becoming a clean and sober person. But I am glad eventually to have had such a strong coming back together as a family. We were not divided at all: we had a strong bond and a real one. We got to that stage in our own strange way, but oddly it could not have turned out any better for my dad, because Ireland had such a strong place in his heart. I felt in some way that I was able to reconnect him to a time when he had known real happiness.

18

There was always a clash in my life between what Irish people would call the working-class sentiments in my upbringing and the world I found myself in when I came to Ireland. There was nothing fancy about St Peter's, but it was considered the most prestigious school in the town. Suddenly my friends were the sons of lawyers, doctors and engineers, whereas in America they had been the sons of firemen, cops and electricians. Kids in St Peter's made fun of the kids in the Tech because one day they would be plumbers. Kids in my neighbourhood whose dads were plumbers had very nice houses because all the tradesmen made great money in New York.

It was very hard to compare the two societies and I was not aware of the class change until I was much older and looking back. I did not know there was a stigma attached to being from Queens. I did not know that people who were more educated or refined could hear an uncouth tone in our language. Never once in my life was I aware of not fitting in to any aspect of society. My mother had always tried to give us the impression that anyway we were above it all in Queens. Her mother always said she had champagne taste on a beer income.

But our neighbourhood did not celebrate refinement. It was not a place of soft speech. It was a world of blatant racism. The winner of any debate was the loudest and not the smartest. It was a world of jewellery and cars, with radios that played way too loud and kids who thought they were tougher than they were.

Loads of the kids I grew up with were obsessed with getting huge by pumping iron at the gym every day. I can remember one summer when I came back from Ireland, meeting loads of guys I used to know, and they would have blown up. They would always have real tight hair at the sides and big hair at the top. They would always be tanned (which was not hard to achieve because most of them were Italian) but at times it appeared a bit orange and too bright to look healthy. They were cocky as can be. They would always be wearing jeans shorts that were a little too big, as was the style, and a bright polo or a Tommy Hilfiger shirt tucked in one spot only so it hung out at the back. They would also often have a baseball cap on that always appeared to be brand new. This hat had to be one that was not adjustable; it had to be sized to the exact measurements of your head.

My neighbourhood was tacky, what can I say? People were loud, and in the summer they loved to take their shirts off. We were always taking our shirts off. For years I thought that was an American thing, but lately I have realized it was more of a working-class thing. We did not grow up with the rules of middle-class living, even though we were sold the idea that we were middle class. It was a modern American way of understanding class, because the American Dream was that we were a classless society.

I did not know that the strip malls of Northern Boulevard were cultureless and that one day I would look at them and wonder how I was ever happy here. I did not know that, as a result of my experiences and my education, I would look back on the people I grew up with and wonder how we were all once the same. I don't judge them, but we could not be any more different.

However, there is still a part of me that feels comfortable in Queens. I love hanging out with people I grew up with there because it unleashes a part of me that otherwise lies dormant. It is the wildness that gets set free when you are away from the pressures of middle-class living. There are fewer rules in the working classes.

There are other rules, however. I censor myself a bit when I go home to Queens. I bite my tongue when people get a bit racist or stop myself from speaking against the Iraq War or military spending or universal health care. I can't understand that becoming a fireman is celebrated as an achievement greater than going to Harvard. I always joke with them and say that firemen are the most racist heroes you will ever meet.

I have this routine I do about being in Australia and taking my shirt off to go jogging. I always feel a bit liberated in Australia because I love the beach lifestyle and I love the fact that no one knows me over there, so I can do whatever the hell I like. So I make a joke about how you can never take your shirt off in Ireland because when you do people assume one of two things: either you love yourself, or you are a scumbag. I live in Dolphin's Barn in Dublin, which is a tough neighbourhood; people there who are perceived as scumbags take their shirts off all the time. I see myself in them often. My life in 'The Barn' has a lot in common with my life in Queens. I see these little tough kids and it reminds me of myself and my friends trying to be tough. I think it's great when people take their shirts off, but I know that all my friends judge it as being 'common'. They would never do that. (I never even knew that 'common' was an insult until I came to Ireland. To me something common was a regular occurrence, not a character flaw.)

'What would people say?' That is the refrain. 'Put your shirt back on; what would people say?'

I like to put the question back to people, 'I don't know. What *would* people say?'

I think for a lot of people the answer would be, 'Well, they would say, "You love yourself!"'

Well, God forbid. Imagine loving yourself. You see, that's the problem in Ireland: loving yourself is a sin. I have a lot of problems about the area I grew up in, but the one thing I like and miss about it is this: if someone said to you in my neighbourhood, 'What would people say?' most of my friends would say, 'Who gives a fuck?' To me that's enlightenment.

Who gives a fuck? I wish I didn't. But in my house my dad always worried about what everybody else thought. And so do I. I always gave a fuck, that's why I never really fit in there.

19

It was very important to my father that I got to Midleton as soon as I could when I came to Ireland. I decided to go for the week of the Halloween mid-term break. So, after sneaking out of my cousin's house in Waterford on the Friday night to get drunk with my cousin Cormac, I headed to Midleton, sick as a dog.

Despite the beauty of the arrival at Youghal, the winding road between Dungarvan and Youghal nearly pushed me over the edge. When I finally made it to Midleton, after missing the stop and ending up in Cork City, I was ready to die. But they greeted me from the bus and I will never forget it when I walked up the petrol station forecourt towards the door.

My grand-uncles William and Dick were jumping up and down, shouting, 'We reared your father right here! This is where your father was reared!' They were very excited, and when I say they were jumping up and down I mean it literally. It was quite a sight to see two grey-haired men in their seventies react with such gusto.

I loved the place straight away. My uncles were mental in a good way and never stopped messing around and singing stupid songs and repeating old rhymes. 'What's that you said you said?' There were loads of them and I wish I could remember them now. Every minute with them was a performance. They even showed me pictures from the days when they would perform around pubs in Ireland.

My dad's first cousins in that house were closer to my age

because William had married very late in life. So there was Valerie, with whom I became great friends, Michael, who was closest to my age but quite shy, and Majella, who was the oldest but was great fun and used to take me downtown during the day. Michael was in a band, which was really cool because we got to go to a pub to see them, which meant I could drink. Valerie was into Lou Reed and my summer-school teacher in New York had introduced me to him that summer, so we used to chat about music. Even though she was my cousin, I think in a small way I kind of fancied her. She was quite mesmerizing. She had dark hair and very intense eyes. They said she looked like my grandmother.

The house was old and wild and the fire was blazing all the time. You had to go through one of the bedrooms to get to another as the extensions to the house were quite haphazard. They had a two-tub washing machine, the like of which I had never seen. You had to connect a hose to the tap in the kitchen sink to fill it with water and the other hose went back in the sink to let the water out. They could not fill me up with enough tea and Coca-Cola. They had bought loads of Coke because they thought all American children loved Coke.

They had a fry every morning I was there and they used to get a freshly baked batch loaf every morning. I ate my potatoes 'skin and all' and they loved that because Dad used to do the same. My uncles would then say some rhyme that finished with, 'How do you ate them? Shkin 'n' all!' It saddens me that I can't remember it properly because they said it every time I ate the skins.

My dad's uncles would point back at the estates behind the house and tell me that the Ryans once owned all those fields, but their father drank it all. 'He was a right bastard,' my Uncle William would say.

Cork people love 'going for a spin'. My cousins were

always asking me if I wanted to go for a spin like it was some kind of novelty. It was just a drive to somewhere, but I remember thinking that there mustn't be much to do in a town like Midleton if there was this much excitement about going for a spin. My Uncle Dick took me for a spin once to a little town called East Ferry. It was a really peaceful place and the marina was full of boats. Even at fourteen I was aware of how nice and quiet it was. He wanted to go for a drink in the pub there. He said it was a spot he went to often. There were no more than three other people in the pub and they were all old men. It was not even midday yet. He ordered a pint of stout and a Paddy whiskey. He had a ritual and I did not interrupt it. The pint looked so delicious as he savoured each sip. He said nothing but it was not awkward. I liked the quiet.

It was the first of many visits. It was nice to be with my dad's family. There was a madness there and I fit right in. I liked being around my uncles too, just as my dad did. They talked quite openly about loving my father. They said it about nothing else, but boy did they love my dad. Nobody ever mentioned a thing about my grandmother and what happened to her.

In St Peter's in those first few months I used to dream about being back home. I would then wake up in my wooden corner cubicle on the third- and fourth-year dorm to the sound of other kids snoring and sleep-talking. I wasn't terribly home-sick in those first few months but I was always disappointed when I woke up. Then I went home for Christmas 1990 and the things I missed killed me: my family, my girlfriend, good central heating, 130 channels, a massive refrigerator, NY pizza with no pineapples on it, and of course having a shower without having to heat the water first. Ireland seemed so damp and dark and ancient, and I really didn't want to go back. Those first months of winter 1991 in Ireland were torturous. I begged my mother to let me come home in February, but she told me that I would have to wait until the end of the year. I was sick of the cold-water taps in my dorm. I was sick of the smell of cigarettes and fag butts in the showers, I was sick of being called a Yank all the time. I was sick of the wet walls of the dorms; you could see the drops of condensation running down them. It looked like they were crying, and I felt like I knew why.

I went back to Midleton for St Patrick's Day, 1991. I loved being back in the madness of the Ryans. I felt free again. I rang my mother and told her I wanted to stay in Ireland. Twenty years later, I'm still here.

20

As much as I want to keep this story about my relationship with my father unbroken, I can't ignore the gaps in it. These gaps are filled with booze and drugs. Still, I can't ignore either what my years of addiction gave me. It was through those experiences that I became much closer to my father, both through the shared experiences of the way we drank and, more importantly, the shared experiences of overcoming it and breaking free from it.

My mother had been right about Ireland: it was definitely a safer place for me at the time. My addiction was hampered by my inability to come across anything too dangerous. All of the guys I became friends with didn't really get into drinking until the following year. Things did not really get troublesome again until late into my second year in Ireland when I had matured a bit and started to go out more with my school friends in St Peter's. I began to go on major binges with some of the older guys from school. First we would go drinking in a pub in Wexford and then get the bus to Bogart's nightclub in Rosslare. It was the days of happy hours and supper tickets, slow sets, shifting and fake IDs.

The happy hour meant that loads of people would stock up on cheap booze when they arrived. As a result they would leave so many full pints on the table. All I needed was money to get in and the confidence to steal as many pints as possible. The rest was down to quick hands. Use it or lose it.

I grew very tall and lost my zits, and my confidence grew. I began to crave the buzz of Saturday nights, drinking and meeting girls. In the early parts of my final year in St Peter's I began to get out of control and, for the first time, I had a violent blackout.

In my show I joke about why I gave up drinking. I say that I got sick and tired of coming out of blackouts, surrounded by really angry people, and turning to my friend and saying, 'Hey, man, what is going on here?' They reply by saying, 'I don't know, but it's all got to do with you!'

That is actually taken from a real-life memory of the Halloween weekend of 1992. I blacked out in a nightclub and, for reasons I don't know, I punched a friend of mine from school in the face. When I say I don't know why, I really mean I don't know why. Many times after this I would have the same experience, but that was the first time. I was popping in and out of this blackout; but I remember various people in my face and then getting kicked out and punching a bus, and my girlfriend of the time trying to calm me down and then this moment where I was surrounded by all the bouncers and a few local guys and my girlfriend pleading with them to leave me alone. These moments were not one after the other; they are just flashes in my mind. I turned to Mick Gall, who was a buddy of mine, and asked him what the hell was going on and he responded pretty much in the way the joke says. He told me I needed to get the hell out of there.

It was my first introduction to the chaos that would become the norm in my life every time I got drunk. Picture the scene. People are holding me back. Faces of fear and anger surround me. I don't know why I am here, but the rage directs me. Soon I will be on my own, punching walls and turning the rage on myself, where it is familiar and controlled. Amidst the fading oblivion I will chant, 'What is wrong with you? You piece of shit. You worthless piece of shit.'

I can't say why I was that type of drunk. I have met many who were just like me and many others who laughed and sang every time they got drunk. The pain of drinking brought us all to the same place. I later learned that my dad was the same when he got drunk.

For a short time no real harm was done other than a few scuffles. But then I ran out of money to feed these weekends and I began to rob other people's lockers on the dorms. It's funny how I ended up choosing to learn Irish, because I never had to do it in school. I was able to go to an empty classroom and study. But when the desperation for money kicked in I began to go back up to the dorms during Irish and take money out of my classmates' lockers. While the poor bastards were stuck learning a language they hated, I was robbing their stuff.

A few days before the Easter holidays I struck it big with a wallet of a friend of mine. There was £30 in it. I ended up down at his cubicle while he was trying to find his wallet. I remember playing along and saying things like, 'What kind of scumbag does that to one of his classmates?' It felt crappy but I now had £30 to head to Dublin with before I flew home to New York.

The day before I headed home to NY for the Easter holidays in 1993 I managed to show my very worst side to my best friend, Peter. We went to Dublin together and during a blackout I beat him quite severely. The next day I was told the full extent of what I had done. The other dramas I had created were with people who didn't really matter to me, but Peter and I were two lonely souls in a rural boarding school who had bonded and shared together our frustrations with life so many times. We read poetry that we had written to each other and sang songs in study hall when nobody was around. Now he hated me, all because of this other character that would emerge when I was drunk. I was ashamed. I could not believe what an asshole I had become.

I felt so guilty – but, worse than that, I was worried that I had told Peter how I got the money. Not only was I worried about what I had done to my friend, I thought my reputation would be ruined. I was tormented by not knowing how much damage I had done.

When I got back to New York, I was dying. I asked my dad if I could go with him to an AA meeting. I can't remember how it came up, but I passed it off as if I just wanted to spend time with him. He told me later he knew something was up. The meeting was in New Hyde Park and all my dad's Irish buddies were there. These were men I had known my whole life and now I was sitting across from them in a completely new context. The sharing was going around the room and my dad whispered in my ear that when it came to me I could just pass. By the time the meeting ended it never had come around to me, but I remember thinking that if it came to me I was going to tell these people that I understood everything they had said. I was not married and had not neglected my kids but, sitting there, I knew that booze was taking things from me. I had just lost my best friend.

21

It would take another two years before I finally gave in. I won't give you a play-by-play account of how I ended up getting quite fond of taking Ecstasy and LSD. I am just grateful that those drugs were all I ever really came across before I decided to call it a day.

The first time I took acid was the Christmas break of 1992. I was with a close friend of mine on one of my trips home. All I had ever done up to then was take mushrooms because they grew on the grounds of St Peter's before the frost came. I had taken them many times that autumn as a group of us in St Peter's had become like farmers, out harvesting every night after study hall. One time my buddy handed me a pencilcase-full right in the middle of study hall and I snacked away until I was completely high. I lay down that night, very happy with my thoughts.

So when I got back to Queens for the holidays I knew one of my friends could get his hands on acid and I asked him to get some. It was the best feeling I had ever had. We played NHL 92 on my Sega Genesis for hours until the feelings were so intense I needed to be on my own. I went up to the bathroom and looked into the mirror and I remember saying out loud to myself, 'What have you become?' I then went into my parent's room to shut off their TV. My mother woke up and I told her I was just turning off the TV for her. But really I wanted to be close to the danger with this new clarity in my mind.

I went back down and I clearly remember telling my buddy

that now I understood all music: I was convinced that U2's 'The Fly' was inspired by acid; I really got Jimi Hendrix's grinding style, and when we listened to Led Zeppelin, that made sense too. We then listened to Pink Floyd as we always did, and it goes without saying what I thought about them. 'Wish You Were Here' always stands out for me from that emotional intensity of tripping hard. It hit me how sad everything was in the world. It just made me so comfortable with the sadness at that time.

When the clock struck 6 a.m. we went to the attic to avoid my parents as they got ready for work. While we were in the attic I read out the poetry I wrote about my loneliness in Ireland. After I had read it to him he said, 'Dude, if I had thoughts like that, I would never take acid because I would be afraid I would go insane.'

The main reason I took so much acid was because it was easy to get and it only cost £5 for a hit that would keep you high for twelve hours. The come-downs were brutal, but at that price it was worth it. The main reason it escalated was because I was sick of the violence that erupted every time I got drunk. I lost too many friends through violent blackouts, and when I took drugs that didn't happen. I thought I had found the solution to my problem. Drugs turned me into a nice guy.

I went to UCC in October of 1994 after a year in Dublin repeating my Leaving Cert. For the third time in five years I had to start again. I had to make new friends and get accustomed to a new place and I was not in the mood. I quickly descended into full-blown, alcoholic drinking, and by the end of the October Bank Holiday weekend I was broke, emotionally drained and exceptionally lonely. I had not really got to know anyone in Cork and was relying on my cousins in Midleton for any type of companionship at the weekends.

I began to think about suicide and I remember one day telling my very worried mother on the phone that I was so miserable I wanted to die.

It must have been very soon after that that I rang Alcoholics Anonymous. It was the first time I had made the move on my own. I went to Patrick's Hill, where I was taken to a smoke-filled basement halfway up the hill. I went there for three months and did not drink the entire time. But the problem with AA in Ireland at the time was that you had some guys in it saying that it was cool to take drugs once you didn't drink. So at the start I continued smoking hash, though that faded due to lack of funds and no real desire. However, when I went home that Christmas I again took some acid with neighbourhood friends in Queens. That led to a chain of events in which I was trying more and more to get Ecstasy or LSD. By rag week of 1995 I was ready to blow. That is what I did, and within three hours I had punched a guy in the toilets of a pub on the Western Road for no reason. He kicked the shit out of me after that: I remember being on the floor of the toilets getting kicked around.

The chaos doesn't build back up slowly, it comes back hardcore. I had a good bit of money at that time and I went hard at it for a few days. I went to a pub I had heard all the people in AA talking about as the place where you end up at the end of your drinking. It was an early house and I went there at half seven in the morning and drank there and at other places on my own for the entire day. I did the same the following day until the binge culminated in me getting some Ecstasy and going to the Tramps' Ball on the Thursday night. I went to the early house again on the Friday morning and then the money ran out.

I remember the fear I had that Friday night about going to sleep. I thought it would never happen, and when it did I woke up in the middle of the night, convinced that someone was in the apartment. I felt some of the greatest fear I have ever known and I stayed up all night, afraid to go back to sleep.

I had a simple new life then. I would pay homage to college every now and then, but mostly it was about sourcing money for drugs. I scammed my parents mostly. Sometimes I would get money off my relatives. Supposedly I got grinds, bought books, and bought sports equipment. Of course, I did none of these things. Eventually I got behind on my rent too. But that was late enough in the year so it did not matter.

I was lucky because I could not have been into Ecstasy at a better time or in a better place. Sir Henry's was at its peak. It was known Europe-wide for being one of the great rave clubs, and the great DJs of the '90s like Carl Cox, Laurent Garnier and Billy Nasty played there. So, despite the fact that I was heading in quite a desperate direction, I had a place to go that made it feel quite exciting for a while.

I did not know that many people, and those I knew did not have the desire to get high as much as I did. They liked drinking too; but at this stage, the minute I took a drink, all I was thinking about was taking it to the next level and trying to get more drugs. It was not that easy for me to get them either because I was not very connected. Eventually I found a house I could call at on my own and score without having to go to the more dangerous places.

Soon I had a short-lived and almost manageable ritual of drug-taking that revolved around going to Sir Henry's. Most of the people I knew went home for the weekend. I would hang around with them during the week rather than be lonely, but at the weekends I was on my own and I would get some Ecstasy and head to the club. The ritual was great for a short time until the buzz of it was not enough to tame the beast.

I am so scared. I am scared because I am worried I won't get in. I am scared because I am worried about coming up too soon and getting arrested. I am scared because I am nineteen and I am on my own. I hope I know people in here but I have not been patient enough to wait for the people I know to be in there. They are not going out tonight. But I am. I have no choice. I am so lonely.

I wait with strangers on the queue. I listen to their conversations. They are mostly about Ecstasy. Either they need to get it in there, they have taken it, or they are worried about it being found in their sock.

'No, I don't smoke,' I say to one.

'Nice one,' they say in return with an intense stare with no malice in it. There is everything to look forward to. I am freezing because I don't want to wait in the coat-check line before or after. I am only wearing a T-shirt tight to my skin that I bought in Greenwich Village on my last trip home, and baggy jeans. I am dying for a shit as the nerves and the beginnings of the E take effect.

The bouncers let me through begrudgingly. They don't know me and I don't take it personally. They are emotionless and try to intimidate me only as per their job description. I pay my money to the woman who I can hardly see through a small hole in a wooden box. She gives me a ticket which immediately goes to a younger man and then I walk up the stairs to the muffled sound of deep house that gets louder every time the door opens and returns to being muffled again, but louder as I rise.

I walk through the door and the heat hits me like a steam room. The smell of Vicks and cigarette smoke is strong. I can hear the popping deep house sound and I am immediately coming up strong. The adrenalin is in me. I clench my fists and suddenly it feels like too much. I want to shout. I clench my teeth and breathe hard through them. If you could see me I would look angry, but I am not. I lift my hands up to the sky and skip to the dance floor. It's not a decision.

Breathe.

Breathe.

I have gone too far before and fallen into a scag hole. I don't want to go there. I want to dance. I look to my right and my left, and the amphitheatre that is Sir Henry's rises above me. It is theatre in the round. Wherever you are, you are on the stage. I see beautiful women on every step. They are skinny and smoking cigarettes and they look so sexy to me. I look at their thin arms reaching out across the room and I want to feel them on me. I want to be the man behind them rubbing their shoulders. I want to slide my fingers across their skinny stomachs that move to the music all sweaty and exposed to me. I want everything right at that moment. I don't know what everything is, but suddenly it feels possible to get it. Within minutes the dance floor is much more full.

I dance and rub my hands. I am sweating immediately. I know a few faces and I go up to one of them and we squeeze each other's hand for ages. We share with a look the awareness that we have never felt better in our lives. I am so high now I want to puke.

Breathe.

Breathe.

COOOOOMMMMMEEEEEE OOOOONNNNNNN!

I throw my hands to the sky. I have never lost the beat. I have been dancing since I walked through the door. I look to the sky where the DJ box is and I see the men responsible for the rhythm, the atmosphere. I know what they are going to do. I can feel the music deeper than ever before. I look right, I look left. I see all their smiles, their rolling eyes. They are scumbags, rich kids, drug dealers, sexy girls, drug addicts, recovering addicts, E whores and businessmen. They are from both sides of the valley that is Cork. We are deep in the valley. Deep in the centre of our universe. I am deep in Sir Henry's. I am in the valley with both sides looking down and I feel them all. We are one.

I dance harder and I am oblivious to the performance, but I feed off the people who get in my face and shout beautiful things to me. I squeeze many strangers and I sweat. I feel the bass. I feel the bounce of the floor. I bounce with it. When the music crescendos I feel the rush as I shout, and we all shout and I look around and I am lost in a forest of raised arms. I am lost in skinny shadows and fingertips in lights with cigarette ends illuminating some of them.

YEAH! YEAH! YEAH! YEAH!

EVERYBODY, NEEDS SOMEBODY . . .

They chant around me.

I look to the DJ box as the crowd cheers. He raises a record above his head.

The Body of Christ. We break the bread. We are the disciples.

A stranger offers me a sip of his water. It tastes better than water has ever tasted. We hug.

Another stranger puts her hand in my face and I know to breathe deep and I smell the Vicks and it makes me feel intense. She looks at me deeply and I kiss her on the lips and she rubs my face. I can feel the coolness of the Vicks on my face as I squeeze her hand as she leaves me. I smell the Vicks off my own hand and I immediately put my hands in the face of the guy I know standing next to me. I offer him a sign of peace.

I clap my hands. I can't believe how good it feels. I look around again and I feel I belong. I never want it to end. I splash my feet in the sweat and the water that has gathered beneath me. I rub my hands hard against my skin and squeeze my T-shirt and pull it down. I can see the dirt on my sneakers beneath me and I splash some more.

COOOOMMMMEEEEE ONNNNNN!

Don't stop now.

I tell someone I haven't got any yokes. I ask them if they have any chewing gum. They do and I chew like crazy.

The music stops. The clapping to the beat does not. I can still feel the music in me.

ONE MORE CHOON! ONE MORE CHOON!

I know it's coming. I have not stopped dancing. I am clapping and stamping my feet.

I can't even tell if I am still high or just pumped full of energy. But I am happy still.

The euphoria peaks again as the final tune gets played.

COOOOMMMMMEEEE ONNNNNN!

And then the music stops. The clapping fades.

And then the sound of footsteps.

The clamouring for parties.

The reality that I know no one.

I walk outside.

I am cold.

I am afraid.

I am saturated.

I am afraid I won't find a place to go.

I am afraid I won't find more drugs.

I am afraid I will never be back here again.

On the night of 15 July 1995 I took my last drink and drug. I am confident I will never be back there again and I am the furthest thing from being afraid.

22

It was really AA that brought me closer to my father. The beginning of that process happened when I made my amends to my dad when I was about a year sober. I had been a very earnest worker of the AA's twelve steps when I got going. I sort of wanted to be the best possible recovering alcoholic I could be.

I quite liked showing off at meetings about how quickly I was getting through the steps and I liked to be really articulate, interesting and funny when sharing things at meetings. It was all part of my need to perform and my youthful desire for attention. I don't regret that, because that drive was very helpful to me in those early years and I made it my business to become very educated in the language and skills of recovery. I am sure I was very annoying but I certainly did not have many cravings for drugs or alcohol once I got into it.

I had a bit of zeal about spirituality at the time. I was a real believer in those early years in recovery that some sort of god was guiding my existence. I meditated a lot too at that time and was obsessive about trying to be a good person. I was kind of like the ideal student of the twelve steps. I was desperate though when I first went there so I was not much in the mood for questioning the process. I have no problem questioning it now, but I know that sense of purpose gave me a structure that really worked for me early on.

So I got to step eight and found myself listing out all the people I had harmed and, as was promised in the steps, I felt an easing of the shame and guilt from the things that I had done. I was nineteen and really I had not harmed that many people. The main victims were my parents and they were very understanding about alcoholism. Indeed, it was mainly because of them I was in AA; they had made me aware of my problems early on and also made me aware that there was a solution. After listing all the people in the eighth step it was time to make direct amends to them, as it says in the ninth step.

I'm not sure I was even planning to make my amends to my dad on the day we had the conversation. I have a faint memory that there was some tension between us around then. I was on the phone to my mother and she asked me if I wanted to talk to Dad and I was not really in the mood; but she said that he knew I was on the phone and would be offended if I did not talk to him. Even as I write this I recall that there was a great distance between myself and my dad at this time. When I used to talk to him I felt we had no connection and I felt that he had no real presence in my life. Most of our conversations were small talk and niceties.

But when I got on the phone it hit me that this was the time. I was obsessed with the concept of missed opportunities because I had read *The Celestine Prophecy* (a New Age book about spiritual awakening that was then all the rage) and it was my bible. I believed that you had to go with your instincts at times like this and then the secrets of life would be revealed. So when this instinct hit me that the reason I did not want to talk to him was because this was the time, I just began to make some sort of formal amends.

He knew what I was doing straight away. He had done it himself at some stage of his sobriety. I broke down almost as soon as I started talking. I was walking up the path to the main grounds of UCC. I could see the river on my right as I walked up the hill. And as I walked we just let it all out and it was very loving and open.

After I got off the phone I was crying quite a bit. It was a profound moment. From where I was standing I could see all of the north side of Cork City through the gaps in the trees. I was so into spiritual things that I remember thinking I could nearly see the presence of God right there in the trees. Everything was so incredibly vivid and the view seemed so powerful.

The fact that I was looking out over the city I was reborn in, after breaking through with the most important man in my life, in the place that he had sung about all our lives, was such a powerful thing. I felt a deep sense of liberation and contentment. Everything seemed to make sense. It was what I perceived to be a spiritual awakening that they talk about in the twelfth step. To this day I think it was a kind of awakening in the sense that I realized the power of relationships and the rewards of breaking through boundaries.

I don't have those spiritual beliefs today but I believe in being open to shared experiences and I still believe that life is all about our relationships. For someone who had spent so much of his life believing he was not really good enough to belong, this was a big moment. It was not a permanent feeling but it was the beginning of the breaking down of the internalized sense of exclusion I had been cursed with my whole life.

The north side of Cork was so inspiring to me then. Those years in Cork I lived in an area called the Glen. I lived in my friend's corporation flat and paid his rent of £9 a week. I guess you could say the Glen was one of Cork's toughest areas. I loved it because it was high on a hill. I used to take a short cut into town sometimes through an old British Army graveyard adjacent to Cork Prison and the barracks. In the spring the gorse bushes were full of yellow flowers and I would stop and look out over all of Cork from the height, and I would breathe it in. I had a deep sense that this was where I belonged. I still think of it when I see the red illuminated cross of Gurranabraher church, high on the way to Knocknaheeny. When I first got to Cork I always thought it looked like a cross you would see in the Deep South next to a 'You Must Be Born Again!' sign.

And now I felt not only part of Cork, but also part of my family. Myself and my father were a pair again.

23

It was the summer after I made amends that my father opened up to me about his past. I can't recall my initial reaction when my dad first told me the true story of his childhood, but I just remember being so impressed at the man he had become despite everything he had been through. I also remember feeling a slight sense of shame that this amount of mental illness had been in the family. To me there was something dark about mental illness of this magnitude and I felt connected to it genetically.

Despite being proud of my dad, and slightly guilty for the feelings I had about my own childhood in comparison, I was freaked out about my grandmother's past. There had never been a hint of a darker side to the story. All I had ever heard about her growing up was lovely things: she had a beautiful singing voice and she was an incredible-looking woman in her day. That's what my father had always said about her and that's what the family in Midleton said too. She was in a home in England and was not well enough to travel as she was a little senile. My dad had visited her once while on a business trip to London and he came back with stories of how she was doing and the songs she sang. There was a picture of her with one of the nurses in the nursing home – a harmless-looking old lady.

The family in Midleton loved my grandfather Stanley Bishop too. They spoke about him in the nicest terms and remembered with fondness his trips to Midleton. Of course, there was the element that not only was he a nice guy but he was nice *despite being English*, so that alone was worth celebrating. And he was a big fan of the pub, which suited the Midleton crowd perfectly. They remembered that he got to know everyone in the area and would go off on his own to the pub and make friends every time. So after hearing all this anodyne stuff about the pair of them for so many years you can imagine the shock that it was all bullshit.

The first time I ever saw my grandmother was at the funeral home when she was laid out. She died in spring 1997. My father had said his goodbyes to her while she was alive after getting the call from the nursing home. He had decided that was more important than being at the funeral. When he attempted to write his memoir he began it by writing about this memory:

When I got to the nursing home she was in a very nice room with clean white sheets and a window overlooking manicured gardens. There was barely a bump in the bed as she was so thin and frail. I held her hand and, as she always said over the years, 'Are you a detective that has come to poison my tea?' I said, 'No, Ma, I am your son, Michael.' I sat there holding her hand, the matron came in and asked me where was I going to stay and I told her I did not know. She said to leave it to her and she would make arrangements for me to stay in a Bed and Breakfast that was not far from the nursing home. I went back to her room for the next three days and sat holding her hand. All she talked about was her childhood in Ireland. Her mind had stopped when she was a young girl and she talked as if her mother, her father, her husband, her brothers and sisters and her school friends were all still alive and young and vibrant.

As I sat there staring at her face, I did not see the grey-haired shrivelled-up old woman, I saw her as my mother with jet-black hair, piercing blue eyes, high cheekbones and the image of Elizabeth Taylor. How I regretted her never being able to march up Fifth Avenue on St Patrick's Day with my three sons in their Aran sweaters and, if her mind was right, she would have cherished those wonderful moments. The tears flowed down my face. She fell asleep and I sat there staring at her with so much love, thinking how I wished she could have been the mother I desperately needed all my life.

My relatives from Midleton were going to the funeral in England and my dad had asked me if I would go to represent the family, so I jumped on board with them and they booked a ticket for me. I was still only twenty-one at the time and would not have been able to afford my own flight anyway.

It was an odd thing, heading over to the funeral of a woman who was very closely related to me who I did not know at all. By this time I was fully aware of the story of my dad's childhood. But I had not considered how much other people knew, or didn't know. No one in Midleton had ever even hinted that they were aware that anything strange had gone on.

I knew that they were not very fond of my Aunt Joan, who had been quite stern and unfriendly with them for many years while she was living in England when they would try to see my grandmother and particularly when they tried to bring her back to a nursing home in Ireland. I think it's fair to say that she resented her Irish relations. I was very influenced by this tense relationship and, since I had only met my aunt once, I had quite a negative view of her for years. But after finding out the truth about her and my father's childhood, I realized the story was more complicated than I had previously believed.

On the train from Victoria Station to the funeral some of my relatives got on to talking about how my aunt had dealt with them and had looked after my grandmother over the years. Eventually I got uncomfortable. It was the first time for me to hear all this since I had found out the truth about my father and my aunt's childhood.

Despite years of thinking that I did not like my aunt either, I began to get angry on her behalf. I felt she had been misunderstood and they were not really grasping why she might have had legitimate grounds to be angry or upset by things that had happened in her childhood – essentially having been handed a life sentence, having to look after a woman who brought her nothing but pain.

I was seething, and eventually I said, 'Hold on a minute, that is my aunt you are talking about and I think it's understandable that she might have found things difficult, considering the things my grandmother put those children through.'

My intervention was badly received; some of my relatives tried to suggest that I had no business commenting on these matters. And then, as if I had been thrust back into an older version of Ireland I had been spared from due to my late arrival, one of my cousins (since deceased) turned to me and said, 'Children should be seen and not heard.' This was the rage of denial thrown in my face. I had seen what the truth could do to someone I thought was nice when faced with secrets she did not want to face.

I was so upset I ran out of the compartment of the train because I was ready to explode. To this day I cannot tell this story without seething anger rising up in me. I was upset for my aunt and my dad that their relatives in Cork didn't seem to grasp what they had been through. Indeed, my father had seen this himself and he wrote in his memoir:

I believe in Ireland that my relatives had no idea how bad my childhood had been after leaving them some

ten years previous. Although they knew she was institutionalized it was just never discussed as there was a fear of mental illness in Ireland.

I sat on my own in the other car for a while and I felt an acute awareness of the dark side of Ireland and the stories that remained hidden and suppressed. My father told me later that a psychiatrist told him that his mother had encountered horrific abuse, both physical and sexual, from her own father. Indeed, he had witnessed his grandfather's violent alcoholism first hand:

My grandfather was a vicious drinker he virtually drank around the clock. He was a Jekyll and Hyde and he drank all the profits from everything that the farm produced in the pubs. When he got vicious and cruel my grandmother would take me up to the barn and I would sleep with the greyhounds as he would brutalize anyone close to him including my grandmother. I remember my grandmother would hide money for food, but when he wanted money for drink nothing would stop him. I saw him smash all the vases and my grandmother's crockery where she hid the money. He would be on his hands and knees picking up the pennies, the threepenny bits, shillings, half-crowns, etc. He would go over to the pub with a big smile on his face, giving the impression that he was Mr Wonderful, but he was cruel because he used to beat up my grandmother. In my manhood I went to the Odeon cinema in Kensington High Street to see *The Days of Wine and Roses*. There is a scene when Jack Lemmon goes into his father-in-law's greenhouse and hides a bottle of booze in one of the pots. Later when he goes back to get the bottle to drink he can't remember which pot it was in so he smashes every pot with these beautiful flowers, growling on his hands and knees. That scene was a flashback for me of my grandfather as he had done that kind of thing so many, many times. So consequently my trips to the barn sleeping with the greyhounds were quite frequent.

Another relative came to me in the carriage and tried to explain why some of the others might have reacted to me as they did. She helped me then because I was feeling quite alone at that moment. Luckily my father had organized that I would stay with his best friend from Bexhill, Tony Dadd, and he was there to meet me at the station. I could not wait to get away from them.

Tony Dadd could not have been a nicer man. I had such a lovely time staying with him and his wife. They had a beautiful house and an amazing garden. I thought it was so English. In fact, Bexhill was so English in every way. It amazed me how English this part of my dad's life was. Bexhill was a small Victorian seaside town and it was incredibly quiet. It was definitely not an identity my father portrayed to us much while growing up. By the time we were born he was definitely an Irish man first and foremost.

Tony told me they had been little troublemakers, getting up to all sorts of messing. He talked about how good my father was at various sports throughout their lives in Bexhill. He mentioned too that my dad was a great man for the ladies. I could tell that they had been very close – which was strange, because I really had not been aware of him until this all happened.

He told me too of his awareness of the horror of my dad's childhood. Sometimes they would get back to my dad's house and his mother would be throwing all his clothes into the front garden and telling him to stay away. I think this was during one of her attempts to live at home. It's hard for me to piece it all together because the chronology is so confused. He remembered that after she had the lobotomy he had seen her walking around the town in just her underwear, completely oblivious to what she was doing. He said it used to embarrass my father so much.

The following day I went to see my grandmother in the home. It was a weird thing because even though I did not know her I knew that I was looking at my grandmother. I loved my nan back in New York more than one could say, and here was my other granny, lying in front of me, lifeless. It was my first time to meet her.

There she was, the villain who had only just been revealed to me. I walked around the coffin, not knowing what to feel. I stared at her face, wishing she could speak to me. I wanted to ask her questions. 'Do you know who I am? How have we never met? What else are they not telling me?'

I felt a few layers of sadness. One was for this poor woman who had her life stolen by mental illness; one was for me, for never having another granny to love; but most of all I felt for my dad. I felt so bad that he was not there and didn't really have a need to be. I felt bad for the coldness of the whole affair. I felt bad that not many people in the world cared about this woman in the end.

That feeling was strengthened at the crematorium, which was not very busy. I knew no one other than my cousins and Tony. I think I may have been introduced to a distant relation on my grandfather's side. The names of those she had left behind were read out and I was one of them. I didn't even know the woman, and now I was one of the chief mourners. My aunt and her children lived in Australia. I was only there because I lived in Ireland. But I was a kid from New York who had spent every holiday with his cousins and saw his grandmother all the time. We were all so close, and family meant so much to us. How could the other side of the family be so cold? It baffled me, but I was glad to be there for my dad.

I spent that evening with Tony. He took me for a proper English seaside fish-and-chips supper and we chatted about anything that a twenty-one-year-old and an older man could relate to. The following day I went to London on my own and stayed there for the first time since I was three weeks old. Thank God they left when they did!

When I finally got a chance to talk to my aunt about writing this book, among the many lovely things she expressed about it was her excitement that their story would be told. I had feared having a conversation with her because I thought she might feel exposed by the whole thing; but it was the opposite. I could tell from the minute I got her on the phone that she was delighted to be talking to me. She was not in the slightest bit withholding with information. The only thing she was surprised about was how much I knew. My dad had given her the impression that he had told us nothing.

What happened is typical of my dad. He had some conver-sations with Joan in the months before his death. During one of those chats on the phone he said to her that I might ring her one day, looking for information about what happened to them. He told her that if I rang she should say nothing. She was under the impression then that he had kept every-thing a secret from us, whereas he had told us most of it years before.

But I know why he told her to say nothing. He was para-noid about how she would react to the fact that I was writing a book about his life, and things in that book would involve her life, so he was covering his own ass in case she was pissed off. He was just more comfortable pretending it was just me and giving Joan permission not to say anything to me without feeling guilty. That was very much a Mike Bishop thing to do. He was trying to make her feel like he had nothing to do with it . . . even posthumously. However, it turns out she could not be happier and is more than ready to unleash the truth.

Joan confirmed that my father exaggerated the amount of time he spent in Ireland. It was about three years, and he was back in Bexhill by 1944. My father never really shared much about anything resembling normal life in Bexhill before he was taken from his parents, but Joan has many memories of being my dad's sister. She said music was a big part of their lives, which did not surprise me because it always seemed to be what my father turned to when he wanted to console himself. She remembers how they slept in rooms next to each other and used to tap out songs on the wall for each other to guess and how my dad used to clean the floor by strapping dusters to his feet and trying to skate on the floor.

While my father was truly happy in Midleton, sadly Joan's experience was anything but and, unlike him, she does not have fond memories of her time there. On so many levels, finding this out filled me with emotion: sadness for the dead generations of my relations who had been victims of alcoholism and abuse; anger, too – I was angered again by my memory of what happened with my relatives on the train to my grandmother's funeral all those years ago.

Then I just felt sick about the whole damn island of Ireland and all the toxic mess that remains unspoken. I just wondered how such a small island could house so much abuse. I hated the Church even more and the continuing atmosphere of silence. I loved the fact that my aunt and I were going to shout right through this toxic silence.

Most of all, I felt so proud of the two of them. My dad survived the darkest secrets there could be. The fact that they went on to have the lives that they did is nothing short of miraculous. They broke free of generations of shame and silence and did not pass it on to us. Two wonderful parents, who brought their children up free of abuse. That is some achievement.

24

Sometime in the 1980s my dad had decided to begin writing songs with a view to having them recorded. He also decided to take up the guitar during this time. I remember my mother buying him a plastic-backed Ovation acoustic guitar with electric feed for Christmas. It was a big deal for him as it was a dream of his to be able to play the guitar. It was a very expensive guitar at the time and a lot of discussion was had about the best one to get. I think the whole plastic-backed-guitar thing was a bit of a fad, but we bought that guitar in the middle of the 1980s fad.

As I have mentioned already, he wrote a song called 'Run Children, Run' about kids in Northern Ireland living in violence. Nowadays I think it's quite cheesy, but I know I was not embarrassed by it back then. I actually went with my dad to record that song and the B-side to the single, 'My Brother John'. My dad wrote that one about a brother lamenting the loss of his brother to drug addiction. It was poignant for us at the time because a cousin of ours had developed a serious problem with cocaine and we had all become aware of it.

I thought the whole thing was pretty cool. He worked on it with a guy called Russ Seeger. Their relationship lasted no longer than that, but I always think of him when my car gets really messy. We had to take his car to the recording studio somewhere in Long Island because my dad did not drive. He drove a crappy yellow Datsun: it was tiny, and even as a boy it was hard to get into the back seat, it was so full of crap. There was garbage all over the floor, which didn't really bother me, but I remember thinking it was really strange to have to rest my feet on top of old cigarette packets and soda cans. Nowadays, when I am on tour and I toss another empty Diet Coke bottle or Red Bull can into the back while driving, I think of the great tradition of sloppy artists I have joined. He was the only one of my dad's friends who was not married, so it was my little glimpse into the bachelor life which I have now perfected myself.

It was a long day in the studio and in the end I went to sleep on the floor underneath the smoke that had built up, but I always thought it was really cool to be there amidst all the equipment and musicians. There was a woman with a beautiful voice who did the female vocals and it usually took her one take to get things down. It took my dad quite a few takes, and I could tell he was driving everybody crazy. He was terrible at remembering lines all his life. I think that is why he was so great off the cuff. (Aidan thinks he was undiagnosed dyslexic.) But these people were all session musicians and my dad was just a chancer with a lot of heart who had singlehandedly got this thing off the ground. In the end they got it down.

As a result of the success of 'Run Children, Run', my father was determined to write more songs, and eventually it led him to write a musical. He wanted to write a musical about Irish immigration to the United States and he called it *In the Footsteps of Annie Moore*. Annie Moore was the first woman to be processed through Ellis Island and she had left from Cobh.

My father became obsessed with this musical, and it began to drive us all crazy. I won't dwell on the annoying schemes and scams he tried to pull to get somebody to fund it; and I won't dwell on the weird get-togethers my dad would have at home with various people who were helping him write the dialogue. The songs were never that bad. Ed Torres was the fella who used to write the songs with him. They were an unlikely pair, though. Ed was a Puerto Rican from the projects of the Lower East Side known as Alphabet City. He seemed a strange partner to write songs like 'I'm in the land where my roots are from' about a girl who goes back to Ireland to trace her roots. 'When you trace back your roots it's like being reborn' was one of the lines. I know how much Irish people hate all that stuff; but their partnership worked and they wrote a hell of a lot of songs together. Though I was never crazy about the song 'Land of my Roots', Ed sang it at my dad's funeral and it was the highlight of the day for me because my dad loved his music.

The thing that made us all uncomfortable was the way the musical took over his life. My mother told me later that it became a massive strain on their relationship. All his free time was taken up with it. On one level he really thought he was on to a winner; he really thought he could write a hit Broadway musical. I admire that. But his obsession with it lay even deeper than his hunger for success; when I discovered his childhood past I began to understand why he had become consumed by it. He would often sit in his chair with his head-phones on, rewinding the cassette tape over and over again, listening to the songs. He would pump his fist and get very passionate at times. One thing I must say though was that he had a lovely singing voice. That part wasn't embarrassing. The fist-pumping and the humming to himself while others were around was.

The problem was that the story had its foundations in fantasies that were lying deep in his mind, about both his life and his desires. It is the story of a boy called Michael Ryan who had to emigrate from Cork to England with his mother after their father died. It inspired a song, 'No Irish Need Apply', about the horrible treatment of Irish immigrants in

London. That horrible treatment motivates them to get a boat to New York to start a new life. Unfortunately for Michael, his mother is turned back at Ellis Island because she has TB. Michael is then raised by Ned, a kind man they had met on the boat. Together they sing 'With these bare hands I will build my dream'. Michael eventually becomes a very rich man in the building industry. He achieves these riches by dubious means and it becomes a morality tale about how Michael's greed destroys all his relationships. Eventually one of Michael's corner-cutting decisions on a building site kills Ned in an accident. This is his rock-bottom as he kills the man who raised him in a desire to make more money. Redemption comes from his daughter reconnecting with her Irish roots and Michael becoming a philanthropist.

I won't ridicule the story, but within this morality tale were songs about Irish history, quasi-Irish-American republicanism, comedy about cockney slang, the Great Depression, World War II, and even one about the Holocaust. It also has these recurring characters called 'spriggins', who are like little fairies reminding people that Michael is haunted by an evil force that motivates his behaviour. It was way too ambitious – like Forrest Gump meets Darby O'Gill and the Little People.

He had some readings, and it was never dismissed outright as people could see something appealing in the epic journey of an Irish-American man. But no one could ever make sense of what motivated Michael Ryan to be the way he was. My dad tried to say he was motivated by how the family had been treated in England, but it was not good enough. The show was just a series of set pieces trying to tell the story of history, Irish America and greed, sprinkled with my dad's romantic view of Ireland as the place where none of this evil would exist.

Eventually, after many attempts, my dad parked the musical and his obsession eased. He did not really come back to it until the last few years of his life. But these fantasies were ever present. When he went about writing his memoir he concocted an entire childhood in London rather than Bexhill so he could place himself among the bombings there. He wanted to be part of that. My Aunt Joan broke down laughing when I asked her recently if she remembered living in London. He also wanted to tell the story of 'No Irish Need Apply' in relation to his own life. He tried to suggest that while his dad was off fighting in the war, himself and his mother were turned away from places with the sign on the door reading 'No Irish Need Apply'.

That's the odd thing. The musical was not truth. But then, when he came to writing the truth about his life, he inserted the musical into his story. His narrative was evolving even further. He was moving deeper into fantasy.

25

My dad expressed a lot of his discontent as regret. My mother has reminded me that it was not really regret. It was never so much that he regretted giving up the life in 1977. It was more that he never felt he had achieved enough. Despite having been a very successful model for all those years, he never saw that as good enough. In his mind, being an actor was nobler. He had it in his head that acting success would have somehow made him a better person.

My mother told me that some of the acting crowd, the Chelsea set that my dad hung around with, always belittled him because he was a model. My mother saw that they were just bitter and jealous of my dad because he was charming and good looking. These men never got much work, but in the pub they talked a good show about everything they were doing; the pub was where they spent most of their time. My dad was working all the time as a model and making loads of money. But he ended up focusing on the fact that they saw him as less than them.

My dad never expressed his insecurities through bitterness and belittlement like some of these guys did. He just internalized it and tried to find a way to feel like he had done enough with his life. I can understand that feeling: I know that I have the same thing in me as my dad on this front. I am often drawn to trying to prove myself to people who quite often are toxic to me. I have often been motivated to succeed so I could officially be good enough in the eyes of others. Still, to this day it hasn't worked, of course, and in the end all my successes and all my dad's successes brought only temporary respite from that creeping feeling of inadequacy.

My dad spent his early adulthood trying to be accepted by these guys. He would spend his later life watching CNBC all day on his days off and wishing he had earned more money. More worryingly, he would try to play the stock market, based on information coming from the TV. You are always the last to know by the time it gets on TV, and he often lost money doing this. He always told me about missed opportunities when he could have made loads of money. He was fascinated by how his Uncle William had managed to crawl out from under the burden of debt his father – my father's grandfather – had left his family.

> He had petrol pumps installed to replace the forge and he purchased a licence from the post office for ten shillings which gave him the right to haul livestock all over Ireland. He then purchased a lorry and a taxi, and he had a contract to drive the nuns wherever they wanted to go. What with fattening the pigs for sale, he still had a few fields left on the farm to raise cattle and horses.
>
> My uncles were cattle-dealers at heart. They were always looking to beat down the price when they went out into the countryside to buy cattle.

Eamon Doran, the bar-owner, was a well-known and quite wealthy man and one of my dad's great friends. My father would often tell stories about how he could have got into the bar trade in New York. Again he felt that his nine-to-five life was not as successful as Eamon's. He saw his friend's life as more attractive than his own.

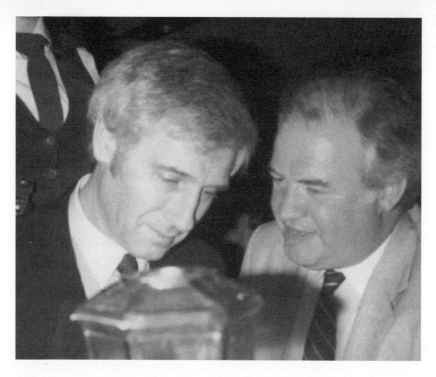

My dad with Eamon Doran. Eamon was an amazing godfather and was always really generous at communion, confirmation and the big birthdays. He showed up in Blackrock College on my eighteenth birthday and gave me £100, a dangerous thing to get on the day you can drink legally.

He would always tell the story about how he loaned Eamon money he had saved up from modelling to open his first pub in New York. 'I loaned Eamon the money and he went on to become a millionaire with pubs all over New York. But you know, he was dead at sixty. I made the right decisions, I suppose.' Most of these thoughts finished with 'I suppose' for my dad. I suppose he was not sure about his decisions at all.

My father would never believe that anything myself and my brothers achieved was any good until someone else told him so. When we played sports when we were younger, it was always about the guy who played better and not about how you played. He would only praise you by telling you what some other father had said about your performance. Early in my career, until he met Richard my agent, he did not believe me when I told him things were going well. It was always that way with my dad. It was never good enough until somebody else acknowledged it. All our conversations would go like this:

'Hey, man, how did the show go last night?'

'Good, man.'

'Was there anyone there?'

'I told you that the whole tour is sold out.'

'Did they enjoy it?'

'Yeah, Dad, I told you it was good.'

'What did Richard think of it? Did he say it was good?'

'Yeah, Dad, he was happy.'

'Oh well, that's good that Richard was there.'

Another classic of my dad's would be:

'Hey, man, when is your run in Vicar Street finishing up?'

'I have a few more weekends to go.'

'How many will that be then when you are done?'

'It will be forty-three sold-out nights.'

'And how many did you say Tommy Tiernan did the last time?'

Even then it did not stop him constantly reminding me that it could all be gone tomorrow. He loved telling me about how fickle the entertainment game was. I suppose there was a part of him that wanted to feel like he had something to offer in that department, seeing as (to a certain extent) he had been there. But really, all he had to offer was fear. That is not a total criticism, and I think that is often how parents deal with affairs related to their children. In some ways it is beautifully annoying that they would try to protect you in that way.

But it was deeper than that with my dad. I felt in some way he did not want me to end up like him. He did not want me sitting around watching CNBC and wondering what I had done wrong, and he didn't want me to have to worry about money at sixty years of age. He did not want me to feel inadequate about what I had achieved when I was in his shoes. He did not want me to have a life of wishes that had expired. He hadn't completely let go of the fact that he had been in the game. He always used to say, any time Michael Caine came on the TV, that he was lucky. When I came back from Ireland all buzzed up about *The Field* with Richard Harris, we all sat down to watch it. My father dismissed Richard Harris's performance straight away. He had been friendly with his brother, so I guess he couldn't give him the satisfaction. He was thinking, 'That could have been me.' I suppose.

To give an example of how this affected me, for years after I had achieved success in Ireland I refused to do work outside of Ireland. I did this because I thought I would be repeating what my dad did when he left London to go to New York. He always felt he would have achieved more if he had not done that. I did not want to look back and think I'd let the whole thing fade away in Ireland, the same way my dad did. I sometimes began to feel that I was fighting a losing battle against my destiny and that it was inevitable that I would repeat the sins of my father. Really, though, it was just plain fear. I take responsibility for that fear; I don't blame my father. I believe that our fears manifested themselves in similar ways, and what we were and are afraid of is pretty much the same: the final truth that we are not good enough.

He was desperate for acceptance. That's a feeling I recognize. So much of his early life was filled with rejection that it is no surprise that in the end he would never feel like he fit in. It is hard to find a sense of belonging when you were forced not to belong in your own home. I can only imagine somewhere deep within him was a nagging sense that he had deserved the life that was dealt him. It's hard to feel worth much when you experience the trauma he did when he was a boy.

26

For years I wanted to tell the story of how my dad's life was revealed to me. I really wanted to chart my own understanding of my dad, an understanding that had evolved dramatically over the years.

The moment that really prompted me to want to tell his story came years ago after I had become a performer myself. In a sense I had followed in my father's footsteps. I know that he was always delighted that I did that, but he could not stop himself from pushing all of his fears about his own disappointments on to me. He did not want me to make the same mistakes he had made. This is a very nurturing thing, but I also think that my decision to become a performer sparked off a powerful force within him. It certainly inspired him to express to me strong feelings about his decisions in life.

In 2003 I made a documentary series with director Mike Casey about living on minimum wage. It was called *The Des Bishop Work Experience* and it aired in February 2004 on what was then RTÉ Network 2. It was hugely successful and it completely changed my life.

It was a very exciting time and it was great to be able to send all the reviews back home to my parents. They were very excited about it all. Of course, my father very quickly began to remind me that I needed to save all the money because the success would not last forever. Then one day we had a conversation I will never forget. We must have been talking about my career as usual and he gave me this bit of advice: 'The most important thing for you is that you never give up performing on the stage. No matter what happens, you keep doing what you love. You don't want to be left with the regrets that I have lived with my whole life for giving up on performing.'

By the time my dad told me about his regrets, I had a much better understanding of him, but I resented his regrets intensely, and this resentment was strengthened by the fact that by this stage in our relationship we were very close. We were both sober men who once struggled with alcohol. We were both members of AA. We were both at times employees of Burberrys. We were both men who knew the unstable world of performing for a living. My dad was my friend by now. I had apologized to him for the madness of my youth and we had become adult mates, free from the wreckage of our pasts. When I say 'our pasts', I mean the past of our lives together. My father was not free from the fantasies that haunted him.

When he warned me not to end up with the same regrets as he had, I did not think much about it, but over the years it bugged me: all these years later he still felt discontent about what he had achieved in our lifetime together. It bothered me that the life he had lived before we, his children, were born had not satisfied him as a complete experience. I was just sad that towards the end of his life he still felt he had not achieved enough. I knew that it meant he felt he was not good enough as a person. I knew he looked around at his existence and wondered how he had got there.

I think my life of performing may have kicked off a sense in him of what could have been. Perhaps it reminded him of the life that he had and the wishes he had that had never died in him. Perhaps those desires that laid benevolently dormant in him were stirred.

I knew what he had really achieved in life. I felt sorry for him, as well as being angry with him because he still was lost in a drama that suggested that what he wished he had achieved was greater than what he had actually achieved as a dad. It must be remembered that he was unhappy with the only life we knew. Even though I often wondered later on how he lived the Flushing life after the excitement of his life in London, I was still raised in Flushing and that is who I am. It is a strange thing to be raised in a place where the person who provided you with that life is not comfortable with it. You don't want to feel less than good about your own life. But that is what my dad felt in Flushing. But that is what he felt about himself too.

In August of 2004 I sat in a café in Edinburgh during the fringe festival. It was raining outside and I was having a bad day. So I was trying to cheer myself up by coming up with ideas for shows. I wrote down in my notebook, 'My dad was nearly James Bond'. I decided I wanted to write a dramatic one-man show about the way my dad's life was revealed to me. I wanted to include all the humour of our relationship in my younger days and his acting past. I would tell the story of him nearly being James Bond and would show funny clips from *Zulu* and *The Day of the Triffids* and how we ended up using them against him. I would then say those lines at the end of the first part: 'You don't want to be left with the regrets that I have lived with my whole life.' He regretted giving up acting to give us the stable life. He regretted not being James Bond the hero.

I was then going to reveal what he had told me in 1996 about the real story of his life. It was not going to be funny. It was going to be horrific. I was going to turn him into being the hero for surviving it. At the end I was going to bring him up onstage to get the applause he had regretted not having had all his life. I wanted him to know that the type of success he was missing was empty compared to the sacrifices he had made as a father and the success of raising his sons in a home that was free of violence.

Once I wrote it down I fell in love with the title, *My Dad Was Nearly James Bond*. It said it all. My dad was nearly an actor who played a great hero who would always survive the most outlandish situations. Of course, if he had become that actor he might have been famous and received the applause of the masses, and for a time he would have had a reprieve from the reality that he never lived in a place where he did not feel inadequate.

I was motivated then to tell the story of the heroics of fatherhood. I wanted to celebrate the sacrifices he had made in a song of gratitude about a deeper, more stellar perform-ance. I wanted to give an ovation from his audience, the family, so he could realize that his performance had not gone unsung.

But, most important of all for him, I wanted to let the world know how interesting and triumphant my father's life had been, despite the fact that he was oblivious to so much of what he had achieved. I wanted to tell the story of a real hero that once had an audition to play a heroic character called James Bond. He had a near miss that epitomized his regret. He spent his life feeling he nearly played a legend, and I wanted to tell the world that the real legend was his survival.

When Dad got sick I knew that time was running out to tell the story. It might seem strange that I would want to tell his story while he was still around; many people would opt not to tell such a personal history until after the death of a loved one. For me, though, this was a project to be done with my dad. I always saw my dad's life as having an element of performance in it. That was not always a positive thing but, as I have the same thing in myself, I could identify with my dad as a performer; I could identify with his desire to have life endorsed by what others thought about things. So I wanted to tell his story in a performance and I wanted him to be part of it. I suppose I wanted him to die 'validated'. I wanted his passport stamped in the only way that mattered to him. He still believed there would be someone at the other end to check his passport, so for him that idea made sense.

27

We became a very affectionate family as a result of everything my dad was going through. When I thought afterwards about holding my dad to my chest and trying to comfort him on the day of his diagnosis, I could not believe how intimate a moment it was. I would say that if there is one positive thing about what terminal illness can bring to a family, it is that it washes away emotional repression and awkwardness. We went from being the least affectionate family to becoming the huggiest, most I-love-you-est, most cry-in-front-of-each-other-est family on the planet. I have to be honest: it felt amazing. Oprah was right all along. I wish we'd listened.

In fairness to my dad, he was always a pretty affectionate guy. I think for some families it is a huge thing for a dad to tell his kids that he loves them, but he was never afraid to say, 'I love you.' My mother was not so heavy on the affection front. We were not really the typical American family; I would say we were more of an Irish family.

Our Irish identity meant a lot to us and we tried to prove ourselves as Irish as much as we could. I mean, we were the children of alcoholics who were the children of alcoholics. Our mother never really hugged us, but she had an extremely dominant personality. The main thing was that emotionally we were not really that normal. That to me is our most Irish trait of all. I love living in Ireland and I think Irish people are the most fun in the world. I would not live anywhere else and I would not want to be around any other people, but dealing with emotion is not Irish people's strong point. I would go so far as to say Irish people are emotionally retarded. If there was an emotional Olympics, I think Ireland would be in the special one, which is great because you are a winner for just taking part.

I don't want to get into railing on my mother, but she hated people touching her. It drove her crazy. I have the same thing myself nowadays, and when I am in a particular mood someone touching me can be the most uncomfortable thing. I actually wrote a stand-up show called *Desfunctional* based around my inability to deal with emotions. The premise of the show was that I turn every moment of emotional intensity into a joke. I suppose it's hard to say that I am not still doing that as I have turned my father's illness into a stand-up show. We were not the type of family that really trusted each other with the stuff we found difficult to deal with. At times I would say there was even a coldness there. Hugs were not in high supply, that's for sure.

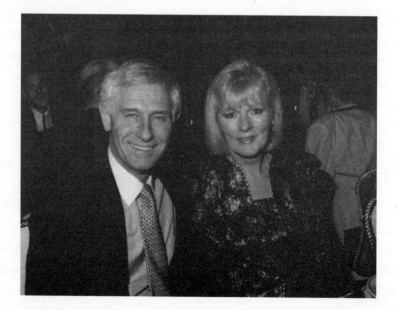

I think the only times I really ever saw my parents being affectionate with each other was when they danced together at weddings. That's why it was so wonderful to see glimpses of their love for each other shine through in the end. I could see my mother's love for my father in her pure dedication to looking after him.

What was so nice about my dad's vulnerability when he got sick was that he needed us. We had no choice but to come together. My mother needed us too, and a wall was broken down by the urgency of the situation.

As I said earlier, I am definitely more like my mother than my father in so many ways. Both of us had cancer before my dad: she had breast cancer in 2005 and I had testicular cancer in 2000. Neither of us went to the family for help. We just tried to deal with it on our own as much as we could. I had some great help from my cousins and my girlfriend at the time for which I will always be grateful, but it never really entered my head that my parents should come over. I did not even want them to come over. I just wanted to deal with it all myself.

My mother was the same. She did not want me to come home when she was diagnosed with cancer. She told me hardly any details about it, and if I asked her how she was, she would just tell me, 'It's fine,' in a way that suggested I never needed to ask again. I feel bad sometimes when I think back, because I actually forgot about it for a while. I never really engaged in it much at all. That is not to say I was irre-sponsible; it just did not seem like I needed to.

I guess in both cases you could argue that we both should have ignored the pleading that everything was all right and just gone in both directions to be there for each other, but that was not the way it was for us at that time. It was the same with my dad. I know it would not have really entered his head to come over to me in 2000. It just wasn't how things worked with our family in those days.

That is why I was so inspired by our time together during my dad's illness. It turned out that we were quite a strong and loving family, and it was such a nice feeling to be there for each other. I look back and see my desire to deal with my illness on my own as much as I could as a rejection of my family. I see the same in the way my mother dealt with her illness. Neither of us has any real desire to be vulnerable around each other at all. We are seriously defensive around each other most of the time. That is why moments like the one on the bench after we heard my dad was sick stand out so strongly.

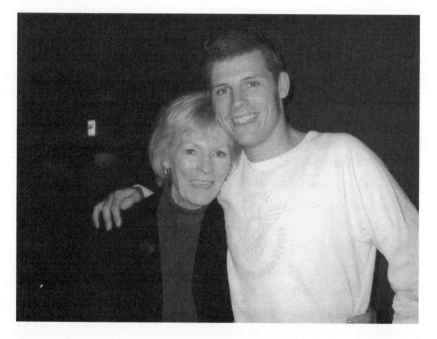

I have been to plenty of therapy and you can draw your own conclusions on what is going on between me and my mother. I have my own theories, but this is not Dr Phil. I won't bore you with solutions or my theories. Anyway, the actions and events are more powerful to me than the analysis. There were times when it was one way and then it was another way, and it felt very nice.

When it comes to my relationship with my mother I would not use words like 'liberation' as I do with my dad. I think I would use words like 'slowly opening up' or 'gradually breaking down'. That language goes for the two of us. It is funny because, particularly in Ireland, I often hear men talking about this momentous moment when they had some communication breakthrough with their father. It seems often that the father is the one that is hard to break down. That was never the way in our house.

Irish people find it much easier to take the piss out of people than to praise them. Sometimes being nice to someone can actually make you squirm. If you watch Irish people in their natural habitat they will commonly greet one another with an insult. That is really a sign of affection. In fact, Irish people feel it is a personal duty to not let anyone get too big for their boots. A compliment in Ireland is treated with the utmost suspicion because it must be associated with an ulterior motive. If it is not, then why the hell would you be saying it anyway, because it makes people uncomfortable. It does not really compute. That's the way we were in our house: we just took the piss out of each other; it was way more comfortable.

I would say Irish people are like the Ultimate Fighting Championship when it comes to hugging. If you've ever watched the UFC, then you know that 'tapping out' is really important. These fights are no-holds-barred, so people end up in jujitsu holds that can actually kill them unless they 'tap out'. Tapping out means admitting defeat and thereby saving your life. TAP, TAP, you tap out to live to fight another day. Well, if you ever watch two Irish people hug, within three seconds one of them is tapping out of the hug for dear life. They are like myself and my mother; it feels uncomfortable, so it's easier to admit. TAP, TAP. OK, you can get the hell off me now.

We can all still fall back into our old ways on that front. I don't always let the intimacy flow. I am definitely a bit better, though, since all this with my dad. In saying that, I am still single at thirty-five; I still find relationships tough. I have to stop tapping out, otherwise I will have no other option but to love myself.

28

It is possible that I have a problem dealing with serious situations seriously. I may have to face the jury one day in therapy about turning something so personal and poignant into a comedy show. I am sure there is a psychoanalyst or two reading this thinking that I have some major issues with needing to share with the anonymous masses things that I should just be processing quietly. I will admit that I always make light of tragic situations. It may be a defence mechanism.

It is also possible that because I had testicular cancer, and almost immediately found things very funny about that experience, that I was comfortable finding things funny about my dad's situation. He found humour in it himself. I think he was on his second day of chemo and the nausea had really started to kick in. He had been getting sick a few times that day already, but nobody had been around other than the family. Suddenly we were all in the room and my dad had an audience the next time a bout of nausea came on. He was not comfortable with so many people around. I don't think he saw it as an inconvenience, I think he just didn't like people feeling bad for him.

After a good few heaves into the bucket, my dad looked up and said with gusto, 'If I survive this fucking thing I am going to get that musical off the ground, I can tell you that much. And do you know what the first scene is going to be about? *Seasickness!*'

I sometimes like to indulge myself in some amateur psychoanalysis as to why my dad was so funny and irreverent after getting sick. There was an extraordinary amount of laughter going on during quite a serious time. Some might say – as I do in this book – that is the way Irish people always deal with moments of emotional intensity: they always turn everything into a joke rather than feel what is really going on. But this was not that kind of laughter. There was almost a party-like atmosphere at times, particularly in the bedroom when he got back from the hospital.

Like him, I was having comic inspirations while I was still in the hospital after my operation back in 2000. I still have the notes I wrote down on the night before my operation.

You see, I had waited months before actually doing something about the lump I had on my left testicle. Then one day I met a friend of mine who had testicular cancer and he described his lump to me and it was exactly the same. This freaked me out completely and suddenly I knew I had cancer. I wanted to do something about it immediately, but it was five o'clock in Cork City on a Saturday and I had no GP down there.

I was back in the house I was sharing with my buddy Ian in Glanmire and I finally admitted to him that I had a lump. Until then I tried to keep it a secret because I did not want anyone telling me to go to the doctor, because I was afraid of what I might find out. Telling him was a good thing. But I was beyond just needing to tell somebody. I wanted a diagnosis straight away; I wanted to take immediate action. So I asked him if he would feel his own and then feel mine and tell me what he thought.

Now Ian is a Cork man from Ballyphehane. Talking about men's health issues is tough enough for guys like that, let alone the prospect of feeling another man's sack.

'No fucking way I am touching you. Are you crazy, like? What if people think we are gay?'

'We are not gay and no one is looking, so what are you worried about?'

'But what if you get an erection?'

'An erection!' I said. 'I am worrying I am going to die, you idiot; it doesn't exactly turn me on. I think I have cancer, the last thing I am worried about is getting a boner.'

In the end he gave in: he could see I was desperate. So we went into the sitting room. I closed the curtains. I tried to be funny and said, 'Do you want to light a candle or something?' By that stage we were both seeing the funny side. And then we dropped our trousers. I have to say, standing there with my best friend, with my trousers round my ankles like two kids playing doctor, I could not help but think that this was, actually, very gay. In fact I would say it was the gayest moment of my life. We had a good giggle at that one, and then he felt his own and he felt mine.

He then made his own joke because he said, 'OK, cough.'

But the joke ended there because he was quite surprised at how obvious the lump was. He told me I needed to get that checked out as soon as I got to Dublin on Monday. I could no longer pretend it was not there.

In the end it turned out to be cancer and I was immediately scheduled to have the operation to have it removed. You have to get the whole testicle removed, which is a pretty big deal in terms of your manhood. People always talk about balls: 'You must have some balls to do that'; 'That was a very ballsy thing to do.' Tony Montana says in *Scarface*: 'All I have is my word and my balls, and I don't break them for nobody.' But now I was having to break them to stay alive. That was a big deal.

I remember sitting in the room a few hours after having the operation, thinking about the fact that I now had only one. Luckily I was on a urology ward. In fact there were four men in the room with me and two of them had also had the same operation. I felt empowered by that. I knew that I only had one now, but between the five of us we had seven testicles. I felt the power of the brotherhood, and the humour of that thought got me through. I wrote down loads of thoughts that night.

I thought about Lefty who was now gone. I imagined that he had taken one for the team. He was like the soldier who jumps on the grenade in the trenches to save the rest of the platoon. He jumped on that tumour and smothered it so it could not travel to my lymph nodes. He looked up at me with tears in his eyes and he said, 'You go, Des, run! I will look after this. We have had some good times. Some very good times actually. You go and live your life and never forget me.' I will never forget Lefty for the sacrifice he made for the team.

They offered me a fake one just before the operation, but I didn't want one. I would not do that to Righty anyway. It's bad enough losing your best friend: you don't want to have to live for eternity with a silicone-filled replacement to stare at for the rest of your life just to remind you of what you'd lost. I really did not see the point, to be honest. I did ask the doctor though why men get one.

He told me that a lot of men get it for 'cosmetic reasons'. Still to this day this makes me laugh. Cosmetic reasons? There is not now and never will be anything cosmetically pleasing about the scrotum. Even the word is really horrible. It really is a man's least attractive feature. You never use the word 'scrotum' when you are having phone sex because there is no less sexy word to describe any part of your body. Tonsils sound sexier. Never once have I been with a lady and thought, 'Hmmm, I am not sure how this is going. Wait a minute; I know what will seal the deal. Wait till I unleash my wrinkled, turkey's gizzard sack of love and she will not be able to resist me.' Anyway, if a girl is close enough to be examining your sack, then she is too far committed to turn back.

So it's not an issue. I would have been worrying about the fake one for the rest of my life anyway. I would have been sure something was going to go wrong. Every time I got on a plane I would have been worried about the pressure. I did not want to spend the rest of my life wondering which one was the real one. I did not want to be buried and then one hundred years later when my grave was dug up to turn the cemetery into apartments, all that would be left to represent me was a silicone jellybean. 'Oh my God, Des Bishop was an alien; I always knew there was something funny about that fella.' I did not want to be cremated so that when my grandchildren went to spread my ashes over the rocky shores of West Cork, the ashes would fly into the breeze and a little marble would bounce down the rocks and into the sea like the pit from a peach.

No thank you. Righty and I will be just fine.

Most of those were thoughts I had in the hospital, and the humour of it helped me to feel like I was in control of the situation. Sometimes I think it is a protection from pity. If people see that you can laugh about it, then they know that you are dealing with it OK. I also liked joking about it on stage afterwards because it was a healthy thing to be telling people about. I knew it would make men check themselves. I also knew that if anyone was ever going to try and piss me off about having one ball, I would have told all the jokes first. In a way it was a pre-emptive strike.

I had just started doing a TV show on RTÉ called *Don't Feed the Gondolas*. As a result some of the papers ran with the story. The *Evening Herald* put it on the front page, with the headline: 'Cancer Shock for RTÉ Star!' It was full of massive exaggerations. I guess the headline, 'Man on TV that We Have Never Heard of Gets the Best Cancer to Get if You Are Going to Get Cancer', was not a great headline. First of all I was not an RTÉ star. Second, when you read the article, it talked about how I was rushed to hospital after filming the first episode of the show. Now it was true that I filmed the first episode and then headed to the hospital, but my cousin Josephine drove me and there was no rush. In fact we stopped at every light.

A lot of people asked me about how I felt about something so private being so public. I guess it would appear intrusive to some. But what happened was that the devil actually came to me and said, 'Give me your left testicle and I will make you famous.'

I said, 'You don't want my soul for the next three generations, like the Kennedys?'

She said, 'No, just your left testicle.'

The publicity was great and I still have Righty to do the devil's work.

29

I used to obsess about not repeating the life of my father. Not just because he told me not to, but because there was a part of me that would not have been happy with it, just as he was not happy with it. I had a sense that I had to do better than he had, just to be accepted. My mother had a bit of that too; she would say things like, 'We did the best we could in the circumstances.' Now I had no choice, as my circumstances were better. I had no excuse for a life of discontent.

One thing about both my parents was that they never discouraged me from pursuing comedy. Once I had my degree they were happy – mission accomplished in their heads – and the rest was up to me.

At times I would look at my life and think that I had no choice but to repeat my father's mistakes because I seemed to be following the same path as him. I ended up away from my family in my early teens, just like him; I moved into comedy, just as he had ended up in the entertainment business, without really having had that ambition; I was well into my thirties without having a child. I began to fear that it was inevitable that I would repeat the pattern. I felt that the by-product of the lonely life in the wilderness brought an ability to get by, but an inability for greatness. Any success was part of the great con job of our charm and personality, but eventually I would be found out just like my dad.

Even in my original ideas for *My Dad Was Nearly James Bond* back in 2004 I had a joke that included my fears of ending up the same as my dad. When the show was over I was going to show footage of two children sitting in front of a TV. The subtitle would say 'Dublin, Ireland, 2022' or 'Connemara, Ireland, 2022', the idea being that it was in the future. The kids would be watching my tiny scene from the motion picture *In America* where I rap in the back of a taxi, which so far has been the only thing I have done in a feature film. They would say something about that being their dad and then they would rewind it and watch it again.

It was just evidence that I was thinking very much about history repeating itself. I thought about my own kids asking kids their age if they had ever heard of the movie *In America*. They'd say, 'It was nominated for two Oscars, you know,' as we had once tried to find a single human being who had actually heard of *The Day of the Triffids*. That was the great thing about coming to Ireland. I used to actually meet the odd person who had heard of *The Day of the Triffids*.

I definitely had a fear of ending up looking back and wondering, like my dad, what I had done wrong. These thoughts were not helped by my dad constantly reminding me that could happen.

I can give you another example of how obsessed I was by that thought. My girlfriend of the time had moved to London. She was a budding photographer over there and was very focused and ambitious. I was really busy back in Ireland and touring like crazy. I had begun to make quite a bit of money and had become quite famous in Ireland.

As the years went on she knew that she could never leave London as she was very happy in her career, and she wanted me to move to London. We actually got engaged and bought a flat together over there. We were due to get married in July 2008. I had some good arguments about why I did not want to move over there, not least being that the money I was making in Ireland was very much financing our relationship.

I did not really care about the money. The real reason I did not want to move to London was because I did not want to walk away from what I had in Ireland lest it should disappear. I did not want to go to London and lose the momentum like my dad had done when he went to New York. If I were to be really honest, I also felt a little inadequate. I thought perhaps I would never be able to recreate what I had done in Ireland. I did not have that perspective on British society that I had with Ireland.

We never got married. I won't get into the details of that, but it was pretty traumatic. There has been a lot of healing in my life as a result of my dad getting sick, and all the things we said to each other, but the regrets around that relationship are sourced from a different place and they still haunt me somewhat. But they are the regrets of life experience and they don't really sting. I would see them more as a fading chalkboard of memories in the classroom, reminding me how not to do things if I am in the same situation again.

The tension in my father was less in him wanting me to have other options. It was more in him thinking I needed to save money just in case. But deeper than that, I think it just made him feel loads of feelings. I assume some were jealousy, pride, fear and inadequacy. I think at times he wanted to feel like he had something to offer and at other times he might have seen me as arrogant and naive. I was on my own journey, of course, and he was powerless; but that could not stop him reacting to some of those emotions.

My dad was like that at times, but more often he was just really proud. Those moments of tension were not all of the time. They were usually connected to chats about money, which towards the end of my dad's life was his greatest source of stress because, along with all the things he thought he did not do well enough, I think he felt he had not made enough money. As I said earlier, he was obsessed about it in the end. They had plenty and they had three successful children on top of it, but he still obsessed about it. I really think money was a trigger for his feeling of inadequacy.

Dad would continue to interrogate me on a regular basis about my financial situation and about my plans. It was pretty much the same conversation every time, and I got bored and annoyed, having to verify to him that everything was going well every few months. He was always also giving me bad advice on that front. He was very impressionable with that stuff, and his CNBC advice was always a day late and a dollar short. Once in 2000 he insisted that I had to get out of bank shares – this was in the old days, when bank shares were worth something – and put my money into technology shares. So I pulled $12,000 out of shares in Bank of Ireland and AIB, which were doing OK at the time, and put it into a technology fund. Of course the dot-com bubble burst and I lost it all. Within a year the bank shares were worth nearly 50 per cent more than they had been.

I had a few fights with him about it over the years. It is hard not to sound arrogant, but I had already saved more money than he had saved in his lifetime. At the age of thirty-three, I had nearly as much in my pension as he had in his pension on retirement. I had plenty of other savings too, and I wished he would just be my friend and not a dad who was uncomfortable with his son's success.

We would even discuss the ideas behind *My Dad Was Nearly James Bond* from time to time and I would argue with him that he did not believe his achievements as a father and a man were good enough. By the time he got sick I would say this tension was the only negative thing that existed between us.

And then one day in those early days of him being sick it

was just him and me in the hospital. He had begun to feel a bit better; I know that because he was talking about how there was something nice about all of us being together.

Then, out of nowhere, he said, 'You know something, man, I have had a lot of regrets in my life. You know, things I felt I could have and should have done and it ate away at me, man, but I will tell you right now: when you get sick and your sons step up to the plate, it's an amazing feeling, man. If I snuff it tomorrow, I will die a very proud man!'

It was the most amazing thing he could have said. In some ways I could not believe he said the only thing that was really left to say. It was almost too perfect. But I know that at that stage my father was not afraid of death. If you are not afraid of it, then you are willing to listen to what its imminence has to say to you. My father was inspired by the power of that. He was open to it. I was open to it then also. I told him he would leave behind three very proud sons.

For years I had been trying to write a show where I could challenge my dad about his lack of appreciation for his own achievements. I wanted to try to prove to him that his life was worthy of praise. But here in the hospital was the moment I was really trying to create – a moment of epiphany when he would finally get it. Instead of my show, it was cancer, and us coming together as a family, that brought about that realization. It was never going to be a rational explanation that would bring him to that point; it had to be something seismic.

It was this moment that inspired *My Dad Was Nearly James Bond* to become a reality. It didn't happen right away but it became possible because it was no longer a show about tragedy, it was about triumph. I no longer had to tell the story of his childhood because it became a story about the sacrifices of fatherhood being worth it. My father had sacrificed his dreams of being an actor for us, and in the end it paid off. The show was easy to do then because it was just about showing off how cool my dad was in the face of all this.

I loved that the fantasy of James Bond, the thought that, had he lived another life, he would have been a better man, was gone. Fantasy is an addiction. You need to make reality fantastic, and never was reality more fantastic than at that moment.

I remember not that long after my dad got sick we went out for lunch; it was myself, Dad and Aidan. My dad had his appetite back and was dealing with the chemo very well, so things were very positive. We were having a nice time just being out and doing things, and my father said, 'God, this cancer is great, isn't it? We go out for lunch, spend time with each other, have great conversations. I think this might be one of the best times of my life!' He really meant it. I have to say I agreed with him. We didn't have to suppose.

30

When I got sober, my father and I quickly broke through a barrier. We discussed the frustrations of the phases of our relationship. The day I made my ninth-step amends to him he told me that he knew he was not the perfect father. In the years after that we had a very good understanding of our imperfections. It never got in the way of our friendship, but would still often lead to some good arguments. My confrontational ways would frustrate him, and his fear-based advice would frustrate me. In the end, though, we used to talk all the time on the phone about things. So really when he got sick there was nothing we had left unsaid.

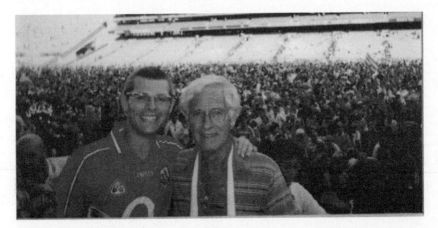

I flew my dad over to Dublin at a day's notice when I got two last-minute tickets for the 2005 All-Ireland Hurling Final. It was one of the great days of our lives, standing amidst the jubilant sea of red, listening to the Rebel Moses, Seán Óg Ó hAilpín, giving his victory speech in Gaeilge. *Corcaigh abú.*

I told my dad I loved him all the time. He said the same to me. The love of his kids meant a lot to my dad. It's understandable when you think that he really felt he gave up a lot to give us the life that we had. It would have sucked for him if, after all his sacrifice, we were to tell him to fuck off, now that we no longer needed him.

Oddly, this explains how the stage show finally came into being. In the first few weeks of my dad getting sick, when he was home from the hospital, my brothers and I spent most of our time in Dad's room. We felt an urgency at the beginning to spend every second with him, because we were not sure how long we would have in the end. To my dad it was like a performance. He had quite a bit of energy before the effects of the chemo began to tire him out. Also, it was heavenly for him to be home in his own bed.

In the presence of that urgency there is a sense of openness, a feeling that you can say anything; but the problem for us was that everything that needed to be said was said. So if there is nothing left to say between yourself and your father, when he gets home and he knows he is going to die and he is full of morphine, he will end up telling you things you never needed to know. And it turns out Dad was a dirty bastard. I don't know why he waited until the end of his life to let us know how filthy his sense of humour was, but he made us laugh so much in those first few weeks after he got home. The more we laughed the dirtier he got.

I have a theory as to why he was making us laugh so much at that time. It is a theory that has evolved from an awareness of what I like to call the 'Irish wound'. It is a personal way of me understanding something that I can see in myself and identify it in others. It's hard to explain the wound without talking about the things people do to avoid ever actually confronting it. But I think if you were to get underneath the layers that protect it – the layers of alcoholism, addiction, abuse, anger, begrudgery – you would find a common belief in many Irish people: *No one gives a shit about me, so what's the fucking point?*

I had a joke in my show years ago about how I was not great with physical affection. I talked about how my mother was not comfortable with it either. 'I am not saying my mother didn't love me, she just forgot to let me know!' Irish parents just assume you will realize they love you because they feed you every day. The Irish way to say 'I love you' is 'Get the stew into you now, good man, and go out and play'. I am not saying that Irish parents did a bad job, I just think they commonly forgot to tell their children that they loved them. I think there is that seething self-loathing in many people here as a result of the coldness in Irish upbringing. I don't mean this as an accusation: I think it's just a cultural norm that has pervaded Irish society for a long time.

As a result of this lack of affection and nurturing, so many Irish people grow up confused about their worth on the planet. Most Irish parents of a certain vintage tend to focus only on what you did wrong throughout your childhood, which can cause you to have a very negative outlook. If you don't feel good about yourself when you're growing up, it is hard to be comfortable with yourself, or with anyone else for that matter. Therefore it's easier to live in fantasy in whatever form. It's better than the reality of not feeling good enough or worthy enough of praise.

In my dad's case I can only imagine what that intense rejection he experienced as a child did to his sense of himself. He did not have to just live in fantasy to avoid being himself, he had to live in fantasy to hide from the genuine terror of his reality. I can only assume having that foundation would cause you to want to be anything other than that kid. I am sure that many times he was convinced he was not worthy of love.

There are many of us who love to feel like we are The Man. There is a sense of being wanted and needed when you are holding court or on a run of great success. I know my dad felt strongly for a time when he was The Man in London. But the doubts would always creep in. He always felt he just wasn't good enough. The wound was deep in him: no one gave a shit about him, so what was the fucking point?

He carried that around with him all his life. It expressed itself as regret and it expressed itself in grandiose exaggerations of his achievements. It even expressed itself in his musical when he tried to create a fantasy childhood for the young Michael Ryan, whose mother was taken from him by illness. He could never face the reality that he was wronged and that he had done nothing wrong. He did not feel that he was worth being let off the hook. The wound motivated so much of his life.

I feel that to a large extent his wound was healed when he got sick. I felt liberation that day in the hospital when he said, 'If I snuff it tomorrow, I will die a very proud man!' His wound was healed when he saw how his family had rallied around him. He realized how much he was genuinely loved. The reality became greater than the fantasy. The reality that, despite everything that had been thrown at him, he was a loving father who now had children ready to drop everything to be with him, no matter what happened. That was the ultimate 'Thank you' a dad can receive for everything he did. He was confident in that, I know.

To have that wound healed must be an ecstatic feeling. To sit there in the end, knowing that you have done everything you can, is unbeatable, and I think that feeling was something my dad liked. I even think he might have become addicted to it, as most Irish men are with good feelings as strong as that. I therefore think that the reason why he made us laugh so much when he got home from the hospital was because our laughter reminded him every day that he was The Man. It was his little hit every day and he became addicted to it; so the cliché is true: love is a drug.

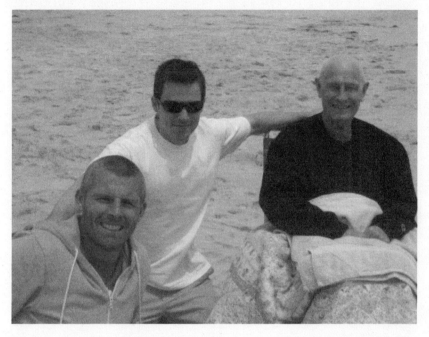

On the beach in Westhampton, May 2010, with my cousin Kevin.

I think he was addicted to it and wanted to feel it every day. He was elated. I think he was showing off just because he felt so comfortable with his kids. His boys had rallied around him when he got sick, so he knew that he was loved. We had mocked him most of his life, and I guess at times he felt like an object of ridicule in the house. Now he was the star of the show and he was happy to take the stage. And man, was he funny!

The more we laughed the dirtier he got. He told the story

of how he lost his virginity with an older woman in Bexhill. It's a total concoction because it has a punchline in it, but we didn't care because it was just funny that he was telling us. He told us various stories about things that used to make him run to a hiding spot and jerk off. It sounds crude, but it was just great to see the guy not giving a shit. We just became four lads talking dirty like teenagers. The dirtier he got, the more we laughed.

Then one day we must have been laughing too much, because he told us the story that began the process of his life turning into a stand-up show. My brother's friend Pete was over and the five of us were up in Dad's room. My dad was at it again with the stories and we were all laughing a lot. He was telling us stories of what himself and his mates got up to back in the day. Pete loves to mess around, so there was a real atmosphere in the room. My dad must have felt it and was on a roll and, out of nowhere, he said to us, 'And one day we wanked off a dog!'

Without doubt this was the most my dad had ever made me laugh in my life. It was a floor-stomping moment. 'We fucking wanked off a dog, man!' He was loving the laughter. He was loving being the centre of attention. Weeks later, my father would say to me on the phone, 'It's hard to believe, but I have had some of the best memories of my life since I got sick.' We had so much fun in the room over those first few weeks.

Sometime during that early period of his illness I had to go back to Ireland and do a show in Belfast that I could not cancel. I really was not in the mood to do a gig and I had been in Belfast recently, so I had no new material. As a result I decided I would try to improv and mess around as much as possible so no one would complain about me repeating things from last time.

Messing around with the crowd is great. The problem is, you often end up talking about 'stuff that I've been noticing lately'. Well, I do anyway. This is a problem when the only thing on your mind is the fact that your dad is dying and very sick. It had been on the back of my mind that my father's way of dealing with his illness was very funny and inspiring. So, without ever making a decision, I began the show by telling them what had happened. Suddenly I was doing comedy about the most recent three weeks of my life. I was telling the stories of my dad dealing with cancer. It all led up to the moment when I revealed that because there was nothing left to say, my father revealed way too much and told us he had once wanked off a dog.

The Belfast crowd went wild. They loved all this material about death and illness and family. It was a special feeling for me too, to be able to release some of the tension I had been feeling over the last few weeks. The fact that they laughed at the wanking off a dog story was just unbelievable. Turns out it was a common thing to joke about in the days before porn.

I called my dad immediately after the gig because I was so delighted with how it had gone. I told him I had told the story about wanking off the dog.

He laughed and said, 'Oh yeah, Black Bob!'

I was not expecting him to have a name for the dog.

Then he said, 'We used to wank him off all the time; he followed us around everywhere!'

It was during that Belfast performance that I realized there was some funny stuff to tell people about how amazing my dad was in the face of illness. The 'My Dad Was Nearly James Bond' idea hadn't fully developed yet, but I knew I was going to talk about our life on stage.

PART THREE

Storming It

31

It's always hard to fathom that most people are getting on with business as usual when you're in the middle of a crisis. The crisis becomes so all-encompassing that you forget there was ever a time when you didn't have one specific thing running through your mind all the time. For me, business as usual meant that, depending on how my dad was holding up, I was going to Australia for nearly three months with a new stand-up show that I had yet to write. I was due to leave at the end of February 2010. Originally I was going to cancel the trip, but my dad was doing so well on the chemo and had strengthened so much by January that we as a family decided it would be silly to cancel it.

I had been living in New York practically full time for a few months, not really doing a lot of work, and when I did it was just little fifteen-minute spots where I could not try out new material. So I was beginning to panic as February got closer. There was some general stuff that had been floating around in my head that I had not had a chance to try out, and I knew that I wanted to tell the 'Black Bob' story and a few other things about life since my dad got sick.

I had booked to do a week of gigs in an Irish bar in New York just before I went to Australia, and I had to go back to Ireland the week before that for a competition winners' gig for the ESB. I had decided to try out new material for that show as nobody had actually paid for the tickets, so I did not feel bad about new shit not working. The problem was, I had not tried out one bit of it. I got up on that stage that night with a set list that included:

- Twitter
- Facebook chat
- ESB
- Erectile dysfunction
- Black Bob
- My dad's sense of humour

That was pretty much it. There was no mention of either James Bond or my dad's past. In the energy of all the new stuff going well, something clicked. Right there on stage, as I was about to talk about my dad being sick, I told the crowd that my dad was nearly James Bond. I then told them about my dad's acting past. I joked about *The Day of the Triffids* and the Blue Nun ad and showed off that he had been in *Zulu*. Before I had even begun to say anything from the actual set list, I realized I had been talking about Dad for twenty minutes.

Suddenly it made sense. For much of his life he had regretted giving up acting for his children. In the end he realized that the compromise had been worth it. Fuck James Bond, Dad is the real hero. That's what heroes do: they sacrifice opportunities for the benefit of others. We never see James Bond get old. But you know if we did he would be dying alone. That's the sacrifice he makes. He will never have a child to be with him. He will never find a woman who lives long enough to be with him in the end or who does not deceive him. It's a lonely thought really, and not that appealing.

It was payback time now. It was time to turn my dad into a hero. I wanted to tell everyone about what really matters in the end. I wanted to get my dad one final ovation for a life well lived. It was not something every dad would want, but I knew it was something mine would. His life was a performance and I knew he would love the attention. It was his material anyway.

So I told my dad I was finally going to do *My Dad Was Nearly James Bond*. We had discussed the story many times and he didn't care how the show might affect him. He was just worried that people might not think it was funny. As ever, all he was concerned about was my career. He was not sure if cancer was a topic that could bring the crowds in.

The week after the ESB gig I did some 'trying out new material' shows in New York, and my mother and Michael John came to see me one night. It was very early in the process, but they both thought it was great and had no real issues about any of the material.

I went to Australia, committed to developing the show while I was over there. My dad was really into it. He used to ring me a lot, asking me about how it was going. I was showing clips of *Zulu* and *The Day of the Triffids* during the show, so I would tell him about how people were reacting. He was revelling in it, because in some way he knew he was back on stage. Then one day he became directly involved in the writing of it. He asked me on the phone: 'Are you telling the story about me losing my virginity?'

Now, recall that my dad had told us that story during the magic time of the bedroom, right after he got out of the hospital in November. He claimed that he lost his virginity with a much older woman. They had snuck into the fitness hall in Bexhill. He said that she was so much older that when they started he said, 'Is it in yet, Mrs Woodcock?' and she said, 'Call me Gladys.'

I thought it was funny at the time, but I did not think it was true. I may have tried to tell the story one night in the section about my dad telling us things we never needed to know during his elation at getting back home. I know that by the time he asked me if I was including that story, I was not telling it because it hadn't worked.

He was not asking me if I was including the virginity story in the hope that I would say, 'No, I am not telling the story,' or looking for reassurance that embarrassing stories from his life were not turning up on stage. No, he was asking me because he thought he was hilarious and that his virginity story was a cracker.

So I was honest. I told him I was not telling the virginity story because it was bullshit.

'What do you mean, it's bullshit?' he said.

'You have a punchline in your virginity story. I find it hard to believe it happened that way. Not to mention I think I have heard it before, because I am pretty sure they make that joke in *The Graduate*!'

His response to being challenged on the authenticity of his story has been an inspiration to me ever since.

'Well, that's the way I choose to remember it!'

I don't even know why I loved that response so much. In some way I felt he was taking control of his fantasies. It was as if he was saying, 'I am not as dumb as you think I am.' He knew it was part of his performance, but it was the way he liked to live. What I really liked was the fact that he was confident about his sense of humour. He knew what made him laugh.

So from that day on I always told that story. It always gets a laugh because I believed it was funny and the crowd trusted me. I would then tell the story of our phone conversation, because it would put the crowd at ease to know that my dad was a part of all this. My dad was a ham: he never let the truth get in the way of a good story. He was an active participant in turning the final chapter of his life into entertainment.

In early July 2010 when I got the poster for the Edinburgh run made up, I put my dad on it as a co-writer: 'My Dad Was Nearly James Bond, written by Des and Mike Bishop'. It was our project together, and he loved that.

32

All those years ago when I first thought about doing a show about my father's history I always thought that he would get up on stage with me at the end as a big surprise. Seeing as part of the plan was always to turn him into a hero, I wanted him to get the hero's round of applause.

I saw that show very differently back then and I thought he would come up and make fun of me as revenge for all the abuse we gave him at the dinner table. I wanted him to liberate himself from his chronic passiveness. I was always under the assumption that the show would be in Edinburgh, so I knew that we would be in a small, crappy venue so he could have just said, 'It makes me feel so great that my son has followed in my footsteps and had a very unsuccessful career in entertainment.' I was then going to show my tiny scene in the movie *In America* and have him make fun of it as we had made fun of *The Day of the Triffids*.

While we were in Australia I mentioned to comedian Jason Byrne that I always pictured my dad getting up at the end, and he was adamant that I at least attempt it. I began to tell the audience that I was going to try and get my dad to come out at the end in August if he was able to. They responded great. In fact, a review on the website chortle.co.uk said: 'By the time it reaches Edinburgh this August, the show could have the tear-jerking conclusion it deserves, should the plans Bishop details bear fruit. That could give it the emotional wallop to make it unforgettable.'

I eventually asked my dad what he thought about the idea

of coming to Edinburgh in August and getting on stage with me. He was very excited at the idea but worried that he might not be fit enough for it. I was unsure if I was pushing it too far by even putting it into his head. My mother seemed to be into the idea as well, so that put my mind at ease. I ran it by my brothers too, and I think possibly they were less sure about it at the start, but it never really became an issue. The momentum began towards making it a reality, but by June my dad suffered a major setback. He began to experience severe pain in his back as a result of the bone metastases. Up until that point we had kept the fact that he had cancer in his bones from him. So this was a double knock for him, finding out that he was in pain and sicker than he had imagined. I was in Ireland at this time, but it was the Thursday night of the Kilkenny Cat Laughs Festival when I was told because I had to go on stage right after my mother let me know that things had gotten bad. My dad was scheduled for palliative radiation therapy, which offers relief for the pain of bone cancer.

My mother told me she did not think he was going to be able to go to Edinburgh, and I assured them that there was no pressure on any of them to come. I felt guilty that suddenly this was the thing that my dad was worried about while he was going for radiation. I had a very fun weekend at the festival, but I was hiding from the defeated feeling that was inside of me. On the Monday night, when I was supposed to go on stage, I broke down crying at the side of the stage. I could not go on. I was so naive to think that this was fun anyway. I felt so stupid for turning all this stuff into comedy and I felt the whole world was looking at me and saying, 'What were you thinking?' I felt like I had let everybody down by running on this fake energy for the last few months. Now reality had kicked in.

But, as was his way, my dad bounced back quickly after that setback. The following week he rang me while I was in Kinsale and told me that, more than anything, he wanted to do the show. I told him it was imperative that he was doing the show because he wanted to do it and not because he thought it would be good for my career. He very emphatically said that he wanted to do it and then he said, 'I want to win a fucking award, man!' So that was it: we were in it together.

I should not have been worried anyway about him doing it for my career, because I think part of the joy in the end was that he felt he was doing that. I preferred this help to all his bullshit advice anyway, so it was ideal. In fact it was close to perfect.

Maybe I was pushing it, but I then asked them if they wanted to make a documentary for RTÉ about Dad getting back on stage after all these years. My parents had a great relationship with Pat Comer, who directed my last series, so I knew they would be into working with Pat. They had been in little bits of my stuff before, and over the years I have had my mother do voiceover for radio ads advertising my tours, so this was not as crazy as it sounds. They readily agreed.

My dad thrived in front of the camera and he loved being part of the process. I was desperate to find some of his old footage that he had claimed was lost. He was particularly obsessed with an old film-reel of a Condor tobacco ad he did around the time I was born. For some reason he thought Aidan had lost it years ago. To this day we don't know why he blamed Aidan, but he would always remind Aidan that he'd lost the Condor ad. In reality I don't think anyone ever really looked for it – because it took myself, Aidan and my mother about ten minutes to find it. It was right on top of the box with all my dad's old photos from his modelling career: the thing was never lost at all.

When I showed it to my dad, he was over the moon. He could not believe that we had found it. He did not remember to apologize to Aidan for the years of abuse he received over losing it, however. He was too delighted to even remember that, but he did remember that the Condor ad was a hard gig to get.

'God, I went on eight auditions for this thing. They were so particular. But I got it in the end because I smoked a pipe in those days. Yeah, I used to love smoking a pipe . . . I loved pipe smoking . . .'

He then roared with a smile, 'That's how I got this friggin' cancer in my right lung; that was an expensive thirty seconds!'

He laughed hard when he said that. I laughed hard, too. I would later tell that story in the show. It never gets a great laugh, but I always leave it in because it's my dad's joke, it's his sense of humour and I find it hilarious. It reminds the audience that it's a smoker's cancer my dad had, in case anyone is in denial. So I use that joke to warn them that they should give it up if they are a smoker. Unless, of course, they are a teenage girl and a smoker; then I tell them not to because if they do they will put on weight, and that's worse. Lung cancer will get you quickly, but fat is forever. It always gets a great laugh and it goes against everything I believe in, joking about in that way; but in a show about lung cancer, you take the laughs wherever they come from.

The other great moment in getting ready for the show was actually quite a challenge for my dad because I needed to film it and it required him to act for the camera. It also required him to come into Manhattan twice in the one week. The first time was to go to a vintage clothing store to get a cheesy ruffled dress shirt like the one George Lazenby wore in one of his publicity shots for *On Her Majesty's Secret Service*. I was hoping it was fun for my dad, but I was also hoping I was not pushing it too far.

It was fun going to the vintage clothing store; but I think it was a revelation for my dad to learn how much his health and strength had declined. We were walking up 5th Avenue. This was the avenue he walked every day for years on his way to work, rushing from the train to Burberrys. Now he had to stop every twenty seconds to catch his breath and lean on his cane. We were in the middle of a heat wave at the time too, so it was really hard for him. He told me that he had always seen old people walking slowly across 5th Avenue and never thought that one day he would be that guy. And now here he was, struggling as earlier versions of him sped by in the rat race. It was tough for him, but I was impressed and I think he was enjoying it.

We found a white ruffled shirt in Cheap Jacks and when he tried it on he laughed hard. He was singing 'Goldfinger' and shooting his fingers at the mirror. I knew he was loving it; he was into the performance. I felt like we were on to something.

A few days later we went downtown to my friend's bar on Orchard Street to film my dad in Bond mode. My idea was that at the end of the stage show the screen behind me would show my dad walking out as Bond into the gun-barrel, shoot the gun as normal and then, after a brief pause, a black dog would jump up into shot and start licking his hand. This was funny because it would come after the Black Bob story in the show. Unfortunately I miscalculated how short the gun-barrel sequence is, and it wasn't sufficiently long to get a strong enough effect out of just one walk-through. So Ralph Arend, who was directing the sketch for me, came up with the idea of doing out-takes. As a result my dad had to improvise, and he was really good at it. Of course, he would never do what I asked him to do, which in itself was funny, but what he did was really good. He looked amazing and you could see on the monitor that, despite his illness, he had never lost that camera presence. He jumped out of the screen.

Trying to get Michael John's dog Mugsy to jump up at the right time was not easy either. I went to the kebab shop on the corner of Houston Street and picked up some lamb. My dad was holding it in the same hand as the gun. Eventually we got the timing right and Mugsy got loads of meat as a result of his mistakes. If you look closely at the footage you can see the meat dropping out of my dad's hand.

One of my dad's improvised lines was just as Mugsy was jumping up. He said, 'Oh, Black Bob, come on, man, you're upstaging me.' I could probably say the same about my dad in my show, but I was happy that this was the case. We joked that it was such a traditional way of dealing with cancer; you know, getting together as a family and making documentaries and filming comedy sketches.

The first time the audience sees Black Bob jump up, it gets one of the best laughs of my entire comedy career. It is one of the most satisfying things I have ever experienced on stage, pretty much every time it happens. It is so important also because it shows the audience that my dad is having fun with all this. He is not an object of ridicule, but the star of the show who can still make people laugh despite everything. The fact that it is the first time people see my dad in the show, clearly suffering from cancer, adds to the effect. It shows a healthy disrespect for the seriousness of the situation to be making sketches about dogs that you once wanked off, while getting chemotherapy.

It was the ultimate comedy release for all.

33

After a few weeks back in New York with the family, I knew
that there was no turning back. My dad was very excited about
going to Edinburgh. Everything he had done for the previous
few months was geared towards getting back up on stage. I
made him promise me that he was doing it for himself as well
as for me, and I believed him when he said he was. I got my
parents a business-class flight, which meant that virtually any
chance to make money for the whole run was now gone. I
didn't care about that; I was more worried about how my dad
would deal with the flight. But it was out of my hands, because
I was heading to Edinburgh straight from Dublin with Aidan,
who had also become a comedian and was doing his own show
at the fringe; they would be travelling there without me.

Michael John decided he would be able to make the trip,
which put my mind at rest. All that was left to do was to
make sure that the show was good enough. A week to go and
I still had a lot of work to do on it. I had still not used the
pictures on stage yet, so I booked four nights in the Twisted
Pepper in Dublin. It was a tiny room that held about fifty
people, and tickets were free. I put the pictures up on a flat-
screen TV behind me, but I did not know how to do a
PowerPoint presentation on my Mac. I thought I would be
able to connect it to the slide show in iPhoto, but it did not
work. In the end I just clicked on pictures from my iPhoto
album throughout the show. It sounds as if it should have
been a shambles, but the goodwill you receive from people
who are getting something for free shouldn't be underesti-

mated. The non-paying crowd was not feeling too critical, and the show went great.

It was the first time I got to show the video of my dad pretending to be James Bond, with Black Bob jumping up to lick his hand. They absolutely loved it. I really could not have imagined how big the laugh would be at that moment. I had mentioned it so many times on stage as a description and people would laugh, but I was never sure how it would work in reality. But man, did it work great. I then told that first audience that my dad would be surprising the audience in Edinburgh by walking out at the end. You could feel the emotion in the room at that moment. They could sense that this was the beginning of something special, and so could I. I was extremely emotional after the show: I just knew at that moment that the show was the right thing to do.

I had actually broken down a bit during that performance; only then had I realized the impact of the pictures. I decided that this picture would come up on the screen behind me as I told the audience that my dad said he would die a very proud man because of how he felt when his kids rallied round him.

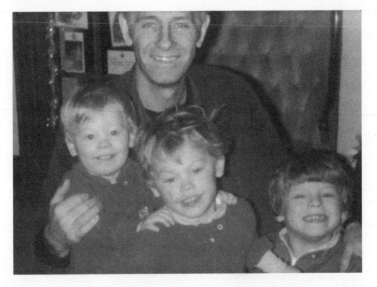

I found it hard to tell that story with my dad's happy face behind me. I could see how happy we were to be around my dad and I could see how he was the only guy who mattered to us at that stage in our lives. Here I was on stage, talking about how we were celebrating what my dad had achieved, and the picture made everything so clear. It hit me that I was talking about something that I felt very deeply.

I loved the show then. When I first started writing anything at all, possibly even before I became a comedian, my dad gave me the advice: 'Remember, Des, Emotion Sells.' I think it was around the time *Angela's Ashes* came out and my dad was obsessed with emotional Irish stories. That was something I used to joke about around the table when I would come back to New York after that. Emotion sells. I'm pretty sure, though, that he did not anticipate he would be the subject of the emotion that I would end up selling.

The show made me feel so close to my family. It was such a fun way to be together in the end. Yes, my dad was dying; but the story would end with us smiling and laughing and, most importantly, together. I could not wait to get to Edinburgh. I could not wait for that moment when he would walk out into the spotlight.

34

My parents made it over in one piece. My dad struggled getting on the plane, as he was so dehydrated he nearly collapsed. The only reason for that was his pig-headedness about drinking water. He moaned every time you asked him to drink any, and in the rush to get to the airport he must have been dehydrated to the point of panic. He nearly got sick in the airport, but he began to feel better when he got on the plane and was able to relax. I had driven across to make sure I had the car to transport him around, so myself and Aidan were there to meet them at the airport.

In the end the entire family was in Edinburgh at the largest arts festival in the world, getting ready to do a show about our lives. It was beyond surreal. It was not until we were all there that I realized how much of an undertaking this all was. I had to do the technical rehearsal with them around. Normally, I would keep them a mile away from my professional business, and now they had to be there. Normally, I would tell my mother to mind her own business when she asked me how my career was going. Now it was her business. I could not get annoyed when they asked me about ticket sales because it was related to a performance my dad was in. Mostly, guys end up working for their dad in the family business; now my dad was working for me. Incidentally, he was terrible at taking directions.

We had some final stresses about what my dad would actually do when he came out on stage. Personally I felt it did not really matter what he did when he got out there. I felt he could have said the 'Our Father' and people would laugh. He could even have sung it to annoy my mother. But we all felt it would be good to give him something concrete to say. I really wanted him to say, 'It's great to be on stage with my son Des at a stand-up comedy show, because when I think of my life like a stand-up gig, then this is a Fucking Big Closer!'

I had always thought of that as a theme for the show. I saw the show as a curtain call for a man who had sacrificed his desire to be in front of the audience for his kids. So I thought it would be a funny, quick way for him to summarize the whole thing in terms of a comedy performance. Plus, I thought it would be a good surprise if he said 'fuck'.

He really did not want to say 'fuck', though, and he had no faith in my line. He loved improvising and messing around, but he hated learning lines. I also think he hated me telling him what to do. He never agreed with me on my suggestions. It's the only thing I was anal about; I really thought it was a good closing line. He got it wrong every single night until the final night. And when he said it right, it got a huge laugh.

My dad hated learning lines so much that he lost sleep over it. All our lives he always got people's names wrong, no matter how many times we corrected him. My Cousin Jen was always Jan, my buddy Mars was always Lars. For twenty-four hours he was miserable leading up to the gig because he was stressing about that one line. It was not really that important for the first night anyway. I was just dying to see how the audience would react when he came out. There was still a part of me that worried that it might be too much.

I can't exaggerate how stressed I was. I had to get my dad backstage without anyone seeing him. There was no way backstage until the show before ours ended, so I had to leave him in the hallway. To do that I had to drive into a pedestrian road and down a narrow lane to get him to the backstage door. Bear in mind that my dad's mobility was very poor by this stage. In fact, during rehearsals we realized that it would take him so long to walk to the centre of the stage that it would be best if I headed towards him as he came through the curtain. That way the audience would not end up feeling bad for him.

I got him into the hallway, drove back out of the lane and found a spot; ran back and got coffee from Starbucks for everyone; organized tickets for my mother and two brothers and made sure they were sitting together because this was also being filmed for the documentary. Then they let us in and we had to set up the show for the first time, and we had all of fifteen minutes to do it.

I had never done the show before with somebody else doing the cues for the pictures. I had also changed all the pictures around and now there were forty-one picture and video changes in the show. We had to get in, set up my computer, get the screen up, check the mics and set the lights before I even got my suit on for the show. When that was done I went backstage and told my mother to grab her seat. As the house music came on I could hear 'Diamonds Are Forever' and I knew the footage from *On Her Majesty's Secret Service* was playing on the screen. I changed into my tux with my dad next to me in the dressing room. This was it. The footage lasted seven minutes and I knew I would be on stage by the end of it.

It was a strange moment, being backstage with my dad. He was buzzed up. I was too, but I was too stressed to take any of it in. The show itself was very new and I was still thinking about all the cues and things I had to get through on the stage. And then suddenly the show began with my dad's scene from *Zulu* coming up on the screen. I waited to go on stage after the opening video, with my dad next to me. I remember wondering how I had ended up doing a show with my dad. I could hear the James Bond theme and I waited for my cue. I gave my dad a thumbs-up and shouted into the backstage mic, 'Ladies and gentlemen, the show is called *My Dad Was Nearly James Bond*. Please welcome to the stage . . . Deeeesssss Biissshop!'

That hour flew by. I can't remember much about it. I know there were times when I felt it was a bit flat, but for a first night it was great, and the energy in the room was tangible. First nights are usually like this, as the nerves are bouncing off the walls.

Then, at the end I showed the Bond video we'd made and it got a huge laugh. I could hear my dad getting into position behind the curtain as it was playing. Black Bob got a huge laugh, and I am sure my dad was shitting himself as he heard it and then his cue. I pointed at the screen where his picture had gone into freeze frame as if I was asking the crowd to applaud the man on the screen.

'Ladies and gentlemen, my dad, Mike Bishop!'

He popped out from behind the curtain. I will never forget his big cheesy hands waving. He was loving it. The audience hadn't a clue that this was coming and they were awestruck. The applause went on for ages. I had walked my dad to the mic and I remember him using his hands to tell the crowd to quieten down. I wish I could remember the particular dialogue of that night, because it was different every night, depending on the situation. I know we had a bit of banter between us. One night he came out and surprised me by saying, 'I assume you're all dog lovers, are you?' That got a great laugh the first time he said it. It really doesn't matter what he said, because it just worked great anyway. It felt fantastic and it was such an incredible moment.

We got backstage afterwards and for me the biggest feeling was relief. In the nights that followed I felt much more emotional, but that night there was just pure delight that we had pulled it off. I was so happy nothing had gone wrong and I was thrilled that the audience's reaction to my dad could not have been better. It was one of many standing ovations we would receive from the audience, and by my dad's final show on the eighteenth night, I began to expect them.

It was a strange way for all of us to come together, but it was also a wonderful family moment. Both Michael John and my mother were in tears as they arrived backstage. Michael John was saying that it was 'brilliant, just brilliant' as the tears flowed down his cheeks. As I hugged him, my father said, 'Tap, tap,' picking up on the joke from the show. 'Funny!' I said and laughed because this could not have been more different from a normal comedy-show reaction. Aidan had his own show to do and was waiting to run across town to do it. It was not the ideal preparation for him.

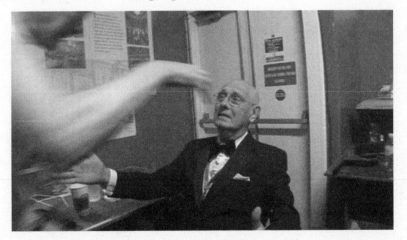

'Give me a hug, darling . . .'

My mother was in pieces. My dad was sitting in the chair, so delighted with himself, but he was taken aback by the power of my mother's crying. He said, 'Give me a hug, darling,' and he stretched his arms wide and embraced her. We have this moment on film and I have watched it many times. The camera happened to focus in really close on my dad as my mother pulled away. It was as if her emotions had swept over him and he was now aware of the enormity of what we had done. You could still hear 'Nobody Does It Better' playing as the audience was leaving. My dad took a deep breath and by the look on his face he seemed to be thinking, 'Holy shit, these people know I am going to die.'

35

The ultimate irony of course is that, despite the fact that we came to realize our father's true worth, in the end he got the praise from the public he'd always craved. People in Ireland fell in love with him after seeing the documentary, 'My Dad Was Nearly James Bond'. I think the documentary excited my dad even more than the stage show. He loved the attention. Just before he died, when Aidan showed my dad the listing for it in the RTÉ *Guide*, he said, 'Who would have thought that I would have to wait this long to get my big break?'

There was a scene in the documentary showing him backstage during the first night in Edinburgh. He was as happy as anything back there, knowing he was part of what was going on. He said, 'I love hearing the words "my dad". "I need a chair for my dad." "I need a glass of water for my dad." "I need a cushion for my dad." My dad, my dad.' I could hear the pride in him then for being that dad. He then said something that resonated with so many people. 'When your children come into the world, I learned that it's no longer my life, it's their life. The only way you could describe it is, it's no longer my life, it's their life. If you go through life that way with your children, you've got a shot. You have to totally turn it over to them. If you don't, they pick up on it, and they never forget it. Children and elephants, they're two of a kind. They never forget, never forget.'

When I saw this for the first time, I was blown away

by how articulate he was about his experience of parenting. It was ground-breaking advice and it was so well put. This really was a final nail in the coffin of any lingering thoughts I had about my dad being stupid. Not only was he very articulate, he also had an emotional understanding of one of humanity's greatest journeys – that of being a parent.

Nowadays many people come up to me to tell me how much the show has meant to them. Also they always want to tell me about how much that backstage scene meant to them. I could give you many examples that often made me cry as I walked through cities and towns in Ireland, but one really stands out. Recently I was in Dún Laoghaire early in the morning, walking on the pier. This man came up to me with his young daughter. He said he just wanted to let me know how amazing the documentary was and how much it had touched him. He then told me how great he thought my dad was. It always hits me deep when dads come up to me and say this. So I watched as he walked away with his little daughter. They were playing together as they walked, and he looked so happy. I thought about what it meant to so many dads who perhaps at times see the sacrifices they are making for their kids and lament the life they had when they had more freedom. I know that what my dad said reminded them that in the end the sacrifice is worth it. Because my dad said all this, knowing he was about to die. These were the things that mattered to him in the end. All his regrets were washed away by the love and gratitude of his family.

Dads always make me cry these days.

My dad never let go of his vanity. I showed him and my mother the documentary months before it was broadcast. It was just the three of us watching. It's always a bit tense, watching with your family something you have made, and it's particularly tense when the thing you have made is about them. But I was happy with their reaction.

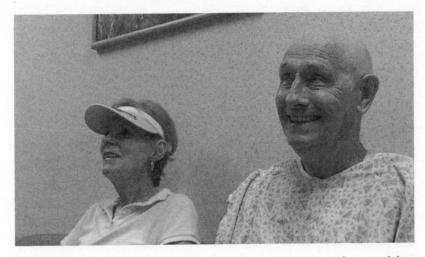

A still from the documentary, showing my parents in a waiting room at the hospital. It was weird watching them watch themselves.

Fifteen minutes passed and my dad waited patiently to discuss with me what he thought. Of course his mind was poisoned with fear about what other people would think rather than what he thought himself, but he managed to get together the words he wanted to say:

Dad: So, are you happy with it?
Me: Yes, I am very happy with it. What do you think?
Dad [big pause]: Yes, I am very happy with my performance.
Me [hiding my laughter]: Great.
Dad: Yes, I think I come across very well.
Me: Yes, you come across great.
Dad: But there is one thing. When I came out of the

radiation dressing room with my hospital pyjamas on and say, 'For Brutus was an honourable man,' that's from Shakespeare. I was joking because the pyjamas looked like a toga.

Me: Yeah, I know; it was a good one. I love that bit.

Dad: But I don't think the audience got it.

Me: I think they will.

Dad: But they didn't laugh.

Me: Who didn't laugh?

Dad: The audience.

Me: What audience? We are the audience. We did not film your radiation appointment in front of a live studio audience. Trust me: it's funny, don't worry.

There are bits in the documentary taken from the show where there was an audience, so it must have been killing him that my live stand-up bits were getting laughs and there was no laughter for the rest of it. The poor fellow must have been tormented watching the thing, worrying why no one was laughing at his funny bits. I thought it was hilarious.

He watched it again after that and he really fell in love with it. He became very happy with his 'performance'. I did not have the heart to tell him it was not a performance; he was just very happy with himself.

This is the story of our lives – my dad's and mine. We are performers. We love an audience. We love to share our experiences with others. At times it seems we need instant validation. I craved attention from a really early age, and at times it got me in some trouble. It has not always been a positive force in my life, and when I look at my dad's life I could not say it was a positive force in his life either.

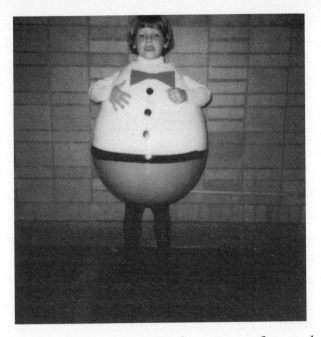

My first performance. I was in kindergarten or first grade and I got cast as Humpty Dumpty. I can't remember much about the evening, but I remember everyone thought the costume was hilarious.

But the truth is that it is also part of who we are and I am not going to look at my personality and say, 'Aren't you the needy fellow that needs your life validated with applause?' It is not the whole truth, because there is also a beauty to it: there is something lovely about the joy that comes from holding court. I certainly enjoyed it at times when watching my dad. It is not like you are burdening the audience with your needs. You are bringing something to them. There is an energy that exists there, and when it's flowing it is a beautiful thing.

So really it is more about the silence. In the absence of applause is there joy in the silence?

I think that for a long time, for both myself and my father, there was only longing in the silence. In the absence of applause there were only questions like 'What is wrong with me?' In the absence there was only insecurity, disappointment, loneliness and the past. Booze and drugs can fill up the silence, but only for a while.

For us in the end there was joy in the silence. More importantly, there was joy in togetherness. I think it is a new way for me to understand the expression 'We made peace'. It was not as if there was major conflict to resolve. It was more like through being open to appreciating our time together in his illness and working together on the show, it brought us a peace that was very deep.

The show – the peace – was something we made together. We brought it to an audience. That is what we do. It wasn't because we needed to; it was because it was something we loved to do. It might also be that we were each other's audience, and we impressed each other a lot.

As for my dad and what he brought to me, it was all about the liberation from the fear that I could not advance beyond what I had already achieved. By the time we did the show I had got over my fears around leaving Ireland, and by this stage I had performed all over the world, but I thought it was quite poignant that it was the show I did with my dad that was the first really successful thing I had done anywhere outside Ireland. Our show in Edinburgh was a resounding success: everyone was talking about it. When we got a five-star review in the *Guardian*, I knew we had achieved something at the highest level of international comedy and performance. I just thought it was great that one of the main sources of my fear and anxiety actually helped me to conquer them. I thought it was great that for him he was doing the same.

I know he was going to the grave more fulfilled than

before he got sick. My mother is convinced it was all he lived for in the end. The TV documentary came out eight days before he died.

A few days before my dad died, I came home to say good-bye, and though he could hardly speak he grabbed my hand, and the first thing he said to me was, 'You pulled it off, man, you pulled it off.' He said it twice so I knew it meant a lot. I knew he was talking about Edinburgh and the TV show.

I think what he meant to say was, 'We pulled it off!', but he was too humble on that occasion to give himself the credit. The whole family pulled it off. We were open to it. We went with that experience as a way to get through it all.

36

The day we were told my dad had cancer and my mother said, 'Desmond, I can't handle this, you need to handle it,' it was as if she was handing me the baton of control in the family and I was grabbing it and running a stage of the relay of our lives together. Michael John was living in America full time, and when I went on tour to Australia or back to Ireland he looked after everything. Really, once my dad got sick we both took on strong roles, because Michael John had also just been through it with his father-in-law and had a good idea of the right questions to ask. He was the only one who was a father, so he already understood the responsibility of caretaking.

But Aidan got his time to look after our dad at the end. Like myself, Aidan also stopped drinking at the age of nineteen. Before he had finished college, he started doing open spots in New York City, trying to break into comedy there. He did not tell anyone in the family, but when I found out about it I suggested that when he finished college he should move to Ireland and help me run the International Comedy Club, a night I ran every week at the International Bar on Wicklow Street. I thought that he would come over for a while and become a better comedian and then move back to New York. He moved over at the beginning of 2003 and ended up never going back to New York. He was the opening act for me during the Irish tour of *My Dad Was Nearly James Bond.*

When my dad stopped chemo and took a bad turn with pain, Aidan was the one who went home and grabbed the baton, and he was the anchor in the end. He really got stuck with the shit job, literally. He was the one who had to put my dad in diapers. He had to learn how to move my dad around in a way so that his bedclothes could be changed. He was the one who watched as my dad slowly faded from coherence. By the time I got back to New York, my father was waving his hands in the air, cheering the presence of death like some never-ending Mexican wave.

Aidan had helped him to get to that place comfortably. He did a great job. It was wonderful that he was able to do that because he had taken a back seat before, which is what I think the youngest commonly does. There seems to be some subconscious hierarchy in his head that makes him feel like his input should come last. But he did it despite the fact that he had to cancel loads of work.

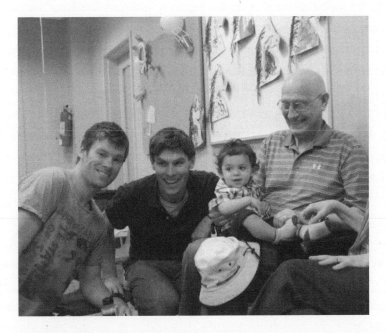

Aidan jokes, 'Des gave Dad a documentary and put him back on stage, Michael John gave him Kieran, his first grandson, and I gave him suppositories that helped him to shit for the first time in two weeks. All of those things brought my father pure bliss in those final days.'

For us this is extra funny, because when we were kids we used to make Aidan clean up the dog poo from out in our front garden because he was the youngest. For a while he hated it, but we used to try and cheer him up by calling him POO MAN as if he was a superhero. 'Aidan, you better go out in the garden. I think this is a job for POO MAN!' It was nice that that poo man got to put his cape on one last time.

Michael John does not drink anymore either, but he stayed out there a little bit longer. Although I find him hilarious, he did not take the same route as me and Aidan. He became a teacher. This is not to say he was not like my dad, because he was always incredibly good at sports, particularly soccer. Sports were always a huge part of his life and he went to college on a soccer scholarship. His sporting prowess was always a source of great pride for my father, though I think at times Michael John had too much pressure put on him as a child. My dad pushed my brother hard but, worse than that, later he held on to thoughts that my brother could have done more with his talent in sport. That was the unfortunate thing about my dad: he saw everything in hindsight in terms of what could have been better. It was as if he was programmed to see life in terms of regret.

The tension between my father and brother on that front was never overpowering and was very much between them. Eventually my father could not have been prouder of what a wonderful teacher my brother became. More importantly, though, he could not have been prouder of what a wonderful father my brother became. I could not be any prouder of those things either. I could go on for a long time about the things I love about my brother Michael John. I could go on for a long time too about why he drives me crazy, and I know he could say the same about me. I love his kids more than I thought an uncle could love his nephews. Plus it helped to watch Kieran grow as my father faded away. It helped to make sense of what life is about. It did not need to be said, it just helped me to see that the journey continues regardless.

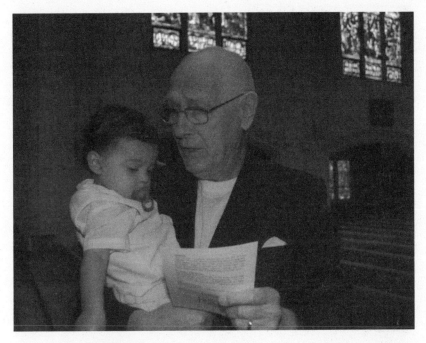

My dad with Kieran on the day of his christening.

Michael John is the only one of us who is married, of course, and I think that is an indictment of the unstable world of comedy. It has never been great for sustaining relationships.

But we made a great team, my mother included. We all did our bits at the right time and we didn't have too many fights. Funnily enough, the only fight I can really remember is the fight I had with Michael John over the eulogy on the morning of the funeral. Of course we were going to clash when it came to the performance. We were our father's children; we wanted to make sure that the audience left thinking it was the most amazing funeral ever. It is the way he would have wanted it, and I was not going to live my days regretting how it went.

People always ask me how we were able to be so open at that time. It is really simple: we just let go. We were inspired by my dad letting go. 'If I snuff it tomorrow, I will die a very proud man!' It hits me even more now, what that meant to me and my brothers. That pride is inspiring.

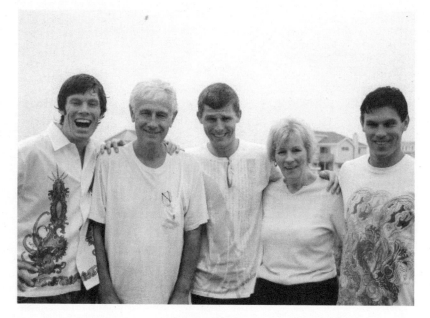

All of us in the Hamptons, around 2005.

It washes away all the disappointment. It neutralizes all those conversations about money. It cleanses Michael John of the stresses of having to be the best damn footballer in the world just to feel good enough. It makes Aidan realize that he does not have to be famous to be good enough. It says to a little boy wandering away from the pitch after walking out of the goals that you don't have to be ashamed anymore.

It was more powerful than any standing ovation. I mean, it was great that we got one every night in Edinburgh, but honestly, after what we did together as a family, if I snuffed it tomorrow I would die with the same pride.

My dad was found out by my brothers and myself. He had conned himself into thinking he was less than he was. He lived by that con and passed it on to us. We found out that he was much more impressive than we thought. In light of that, we found out that we too were much more impressive than we thought. A cloud of shame was lifted from our family. Our togetherness was an inspiration: it was a sense of family I had never really known was there.

37

I was not meant to come home for Christmas 2010; my parents were meant to come to Ireland. The incredible December weather in Dublin stopped that plan in its tracks. My parents' flight was officially cancelled at around 3 p.m. on 20 December. They had been due to fly out that night. I remember the moment because I was stuck in the most unbelievable traffic on the M50, and I broke down crying at the thought of not seeing my father for what was going to be our last Christmas together.

It turned out to be a blessing because he never even got out of bed that day. The week leading up to him coming to Ireland was actually the week when my mother began to realize that the chemo was not really working at all. In the end it was just a fluke that the flight got cancelled due to the snow, because I don't think my dad would have been able to get on the plane.

It was sad for me though, because my dad had been going on about getting back to Ireland and looking forward to being wheeled down Grafton Street on Christmas Eve. He had loved the last time we all did that as a family, a few years earlier when we spent our first Christmas in Ireland together. It was one of the best Christmases we'd ever had. He was hoping to listen to the buskers again and meet up with all the people you bump into on that day in Dublin.

Really, I was lucky that he did not make it over because this time I had been telling anyone in Ireland who would listen very embarrassing stories about my dad. So now it would not just be me people recognized on the street, but also him. They would have shouted, 'Mayday! Mayday!' back at him or even reminded him of the Black Bob story.

When I finally got off the M50, I turned the tears into action, and myself and my brother Aidan got a Newark flight out of Shannon on Christmas Eve. I deliberately picked Shannon because it had not been snowing on the west coast. It was a good call because, even though flights left Dublin that day, it had snowed the night before and it would not have been worth the stress. I was taking no risks. So, on the night of 23 December, in the middle of one of the worst snowstorms I have ever seen in Ireland, we headed to Shannon.

It was a bitter-sweet thing to be home with the family, knowing that the end was very near. It was great to get there, but I could see how much my dad had declined since the end of October when I was last home. He was very weak and struggling to get out of bed. My nephew Kieran's cuteness and development into the most fun ever added to the sweetness. It helped to turn the sadness into celebration.

This was really the second time we were having Dad's last Christmas. I have a picture of my mom crying at Christmas 2009 because she thought it was going to be the last family photo at Christmas. We all thought that back then. It was sad to know that he would not pull it off for another one, but it was wonderful to be having one more Christmas together. This was our consolation Christmas.

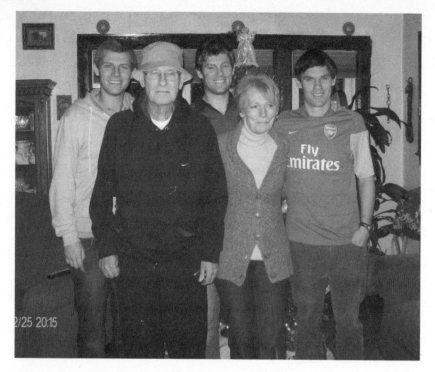

Christmas 2009.

On Christmas morning I was getting my dad ready to get up and take the slow trip down the stairs. He had not been down there for three days, but he was feeling better in the last two days and had saved his energy for Christmas Day so he could have dinner and enjoy the company. I don't know how we got on the subject of songs, but he asked me if I knew the song, 'Dublin in the Rare Auld Times'. He sang a bit of it but I only knew the 'ring a ring a rosie' bit and that was all he knew, too. So I got out my iPhone and looked it up. There was a version by Ronnie Drew on it and I played him that and he sang along. I found it very sad because I knew Ronnie had died of cancer and I know his son, Phelim. It brought it home to me that my dad was not going to be around for very long. I felt sadness for Phelim, who is such a lovely guy, and this fed into my sorrow that I would soon be part of that club. But my dad sang away, happy to be alive for that moment.

Listening to Ronnie Drew reminded me that my friend Cathal had bought my father a Luke Kelly CD for Christmas, so I thought that I could play him 'Raglan Road' on the iPhone to see if he liked Luke Kelly.

While we listened I got my dad's sneakers to put them on him. I had a routine with all that, so getting them on was no big deal. But, for some reason, as I was tying his laces my eyes began to tear up. 'Raglan Road' is a sad song anyway, but just being there listening to it while tying the laces of the man who tied mine when I was a boy was heartbreaking. I loved him very much at that moment. I was so happy I was able to take care of him. I kept my head down and did not let him know that I was crying.

We got downstairs and opened the presents. Dad loved his Luke Kelly CD. We then broke out the flip camera and tried to capture some memories. Aidan put the camera on Dad and I leaned in with my hands and said: 'Dad's Last Christmas, Take 2.' *CLAP!*

38

When we had already done *My Dad Was Nearly James Bond* in Edinburgh and my father was back doing chemo from the end of August for the second time, with less than promising results, I asked him why he was bothering doing it again when he was only delaying the inevitable. He still wanted to be around for longer. I told him that he had done everything a man could do in his situation. He had made sure his wife would be looked after once he was gone. His children were all educated. He had a grandchild. He had been back on stage in a show about his life that people loved. He had wonderful friends and in his time of need he was surrounded by his family that loved him deeply. I asked him if there was anything else that was on his mind that he wanted to do before he died. He immediately said that he wanted to have another crack at the musical and make sure that he recorded the songs he had written that had not been recorded already.

For us three boys this was a bitter-sweet desire, because none of us had much faith in the musical. We saw it as cheesy and a waste of time. Michael John had done his part and had brought the script to a few people at his school who were into theatre. Michael John and I had a belief that the focus should be on the characters. I was very honest with my dad and I told him that the musical was a fantasy story about a boy whose mother was taken off him. It was also a morality tale about the horrible effects of greed. The consequence in the musical was that Michael Ryan cut corners on a building site, which caused an accident that killed Ned, the man who took him in after his mother was sent away. I knew that my dad had spent most of his life wishing he had made more money. It was as if he was trying to prove to himself that he had made the right moves, I suppose.

I told him that if he wanted to have one more go, he should forget about most of the musical and see if he could be inspired by the true story: that Michael Ryan was not on a boat with his mother, but was, in fact, with his 'Uncle Ned' who had come to England to take him away from his abusive mother. The story of his mother being taken away at Ellis Island was a myth that his uncle and himself had decided would be the story they told for life. The story of his father being dead was part of that lie too, because he was never able to make sense of why a father could let that kind of abuse happen to a son. Michael Ryan's greed was driven by his need to feel like he had achieved enough and was good enough in the eyes of society because, when push came to shove, he held on to the secret of his own abandonment and rejection.

The same secret was the very thing that drove a wedge between himself and everyone he loved because he feared getting close to anyone, lest the same thing should happen. His greatest fear was being found out as a phoney. He would go to any lengths to ensure that didn't happen. Inevitably, those desires caused him to kill the very man who had saved him.

The rest doesn't really matter. I just wanted my dad to stop turning his mother into an angel. I wanted him to stop pretending that he was not the victim. I really did not care about how the story panned out, I just wanted him to stop writing the fantasy and be inspired by the reality. The redemption in the story would come when Michael finally admitted to his wife and daughter that his silence and greed were motivated by a secret about his parents he had kept all his life. He admitted at times to feeling so distant from them because he resented the very peace he had provided for them that had been so cruelly taken from him.

It is dramatic and it was not a direct translation from my dad's life, but that didn't matter. My dad was about to die and he saw many things in a dramatic way, and there were way too many comparisons with his own life for that to be a coincidence. Even the way Ireland appears as this idyllic place in the story is part of my dad's fantasy. My father always saw Midleton as a place of refuge from any turmoil he would feel later in life. It was where he went to escape, both in reality and in his own head.

Working on the musical was very healing, and he stayed at it from September 2010 until shortly before he died. He changed the title to *Secrets* and tried to think of the story in terms of the all-too-common tale of the poison that silence has brought to Irish society. He wrote a new song called 'Redeem Me', about Michael singing to the heavens after the death of Ned and the rejection of his daughter.

> Stay with me tonight, Lord.
> Stay with me tonight.
> Stay with me, oh stay with me
> In my hour of need.

Those were the opening lines of the song. He recorded it in his bed, two weeks before he died. Ed Torres put it together and, less than a week before he died, he was able to listen to it. I was not home yet, but my brother filmed my father listening to it. He was already heading towards death, and he looked as if he was being freed to let go. In his head the toll had been paid and the barrier had risen. It had been his final wish to record another song in the musical, and it was so great that it was a song about redemption.

Ed Torres said to my dad in the room that day, 'You did it, Mike, you did it.' He certainly did. I will always be grateful to Ed for giving my dad his dying wish. We gave Ed the Ovation guitar as a gift from my dad after he died. He will always have that to remind him of my dad and the 1980s.

Funny that, despite the things she did, in the end my dad and his mother both went out singing.

39

Journal, 11 January 2011, Dublin

I rang home last night at about 8 p.m., knowing that my dad had been due to start chemo again yesterday after an extended break. I also knew that he was getting weaker and none of us were sure if he had the strength for the fight anymore. I ring home pretty much every day, but I knew that this call was probably more important than normal.

My father answered the phone, which was just luck, really. All it meant was that my mother had stepped out. There was nothing strange about the fact that he had answered. It was lucky for me, though, because I was glad to get the news directly from him; he told me that he had not gone ahead with the chemo. This didn't surprise me, because he was so weak. I did not expect that he would tell me that he had decided to stop getting chemo altogether, though. He told me that he had told the oncologist that he did not see any point and that it was obvious that he was getting worse, regardless. He seemed to be happy with the decision. He stated very clearly, 'I am not laying this on you, I am not laying this on the family and I am not laying this on the doctors; this is my decision.' He said that very strongly. As always, my father's main concern was to make sure everyone was comfortable.

I thought it was an exceptional thing to say, because in his case it was so empowering for him. I actually remember saying very soon after that (but perhaps not in reply) that he was now in control of his own life. There would be no more being pricked and prodded looking for a vein, no more blood transfusions just to have the strength to go to the bathroom, and no more having to go to the chemo place. It's amazing how deciding that you are now ready to let the disease take over brings a relief and a sense of freedom. That's how it seemed my dad felt. He said all the right things. He was looking forward to the hospice people helping him to be comfortable. He was looking forward to not feeling nauseous all the time. He was hopeful he might get a bit of energy back in the short term before the cancer did its worst. I guess in many ways he was relieved that the fight was over and he could just relax.

He told me the oncologist had warned him there would be pain. She gave him a very detailed account of what he could expect, so I don't think his positivity was in any way a denial. He can have no idea what it's going to be like, and neither can we, so I think his attitude is great. Never is the one-day-at-a-time mantra more important than at times like these. When life changes so quickly every day, all you can really know is what you have to deal with today. Now we know time is short and I hope we can stretch each day out to feel like months, so these last few months will feel like forever.

I encouraged my father not to get chemo at all after the cancer started to grow again. Back in August, he delayed chemo for an extra week so as to spend more time in Edinburgh. I suggested he should not go back at all but just enjoy the time the first months of chemo bought him. Again, when he got weak in the last month, I pushed hard that he should consider giving up the fight. I wanted him to enjoy whatever time was left and not spend the whole time fighting an unwinnable battle. To be honest, if he had told me back in November 2009 that he did not want to fight, I would have been more than able to accept his decision. I am glad he fought then, though, because these last fifteen months have been the best times we have ever had together, but I had not been a big fan of aggressive treatment for a man of my dad's age who has lived the life that he has lived.

Yet after all my bravado and rational suggestions about the imminence of death and treatment, yesterday's news was difficult to accept. Because even though I wanted my dad to stop treatment, once he told me he had made that decision I knew he would die quite soon. The phase of hope was over and now all that was left was preparing for him to be gone. All that was left was the end.

This is the part I know nothing about. Up until now I have spoken with great confidence about the certainty of my father's death. But it was academic because I was protected by the uncertainty of how long he had left. Now there is no more pretending and the reality of that hit me hard last night.

I had so many emotions. I wish they were all feelings of compassion for my father, but they were not. I felt sad and happy that my dad was comfortable with his decision. There was something uplifting about the honesty of the situation. I used to hate hearing him speak about living for years and knowing it was not true but not wanting to break his spirit. I felt regretful almost immediately that I did not push harder for him to stop the chemo.

The main thing I felt was that we could have been done with this part already. It seems a strange thing, but that was honestly one of the things I felt. I felt that I was much less prepared now than I was at this time last year. I resented the fact that after pretty much a year of living at home – apart from a trip to Australia and our trip to Edinburgh – I had to go back on tour and make some money. Yet now seemed to be the most important time to be home.

Most of all I just wanted to be home. I did not want to have to ask my family for information on the phone. I did not want to hear about my aunts and uncles being at the house when I could not be there. I just wanted to be home so I could rub my dad's head and tell him that everything was going to be all right. It was so frustrating that I would have to wait till Sunday.

I wanted to talk to my mother too. She had fought this moment from the start, but she had come to accept it in the last few weeks as she saw how it was literally becoming impossible for her to even get my dad out of bed to get to the chemo place to keep up the fight.

I was very emotional and she was not: that is her way. I can only imagine how much more difficult it is for her. Of course I will be there for her, but she would never let you know that she needs help. You have to try to help her despite herself. I think, though, when I finally spoke to her yesterday, for the first time in a long time, I wanted her to help me. At least I wanted to share the sadness together just for a moment, like when we found out the news a year and a half before. I just wanted to be vulnerable together like a family should be. But she was not feeling that way at that time. She will fight that honesty until the end. I hope she will be all right. I hope the same for myself.

Journal, 12 January 2011, Dublin

Phone conversation with my father a day after he decided
to stop chemo, sometime around 3 p.m.:

> Dad: I just want to spend the next few days in bed
> and try to come to terms with all this.
>
> Des: Come to terms with what, exactly?
>
> Dad: Well, I know the end is coming now. I can see
> him. [Puts on Irish accent] 'Ah, there you are. There
> you are, ya hoor, ya.'
>
> Des [laughing]: Sure. 'Put that scythe down and
> let's have a chat.'
>
> Dad: I suppose telling you to fuck off isn't going to
> change anything?

Journal, 17 January 2011, Flushing, Queens, 2.22 p.m.

I can hear my dad's voice in the next room talking to a
friend of his. There is clearly more strength in it now
than those days last week when we spoke on the phone.
It's great to think that some of his weakness over the
last month was more related to the chemo than the
progression of the disease.

Of course, it brings with it doubt about the decisions that
were made. I have no doubt, but my mother thinks now that
we have not done enough. She is worried that we did not
try clinical trials. I am not worried about that because, to
me, I see him feeling better as testimony to the fact that we
made the right decision about stopping treatment altogether.
Anyway, there is no point in talking about it because he
is comfortable with the decision he made, and that is all
that matters. I just don't want anyone in the family to be
tormented by thoughts that we did not do enough.

My dad isn't great at just enjoying feeling better, either. As soon as he started to feel better he was talking about how he was going to go on for years. I just let him believe it because what's the point in putting a downer on things when he is feeling good?

It's nice to be home. It's not that emotional, I must say. It just feels right to be here and to be able to help out. We completely reorganized the bedroom upstairs, as the hospital bed came today. So now my mother sleeps on a single bed and my dad has his own hospital bed that can be adjusted electronically. He fought having one brought home for so long, but now that it is here he seems to be very comfortable in it.

He does not like anything that suggests that the fight is over. He is naturally a very competitive man and he wants to go down fighting the best fight. Just because he has given up treatment does not mean he has given up the fight.

He has new goals to live for. He wants to be around for when it gets warmer so we can wheel him around Kissena Park. He wants to see his second grandchild, who will not be born until May. He wants to record a few of his songs that he wrote for the musical . . .

A few hours later . . .

I don't know how it happened, but I ended up reading to my dad some of the proposal for this book that I sent to the publishers. I really just wanted to know for sure that he was comfortable with the idea of me writing a book about his life. I am not sure if it was a good thing to be reading him my innermost thoughts about his dying, but if I can't read them to him, why would I be comfortable with anonymous masses reading them? So much of this is about his legacy, so I might as well let him know what

257

I am feeling. It's the much more important thing. I read him a section about him hoping to find the spot where he wants his ashes spread in Ballycotton.

'Why must we wait till the end to get to this point? Why must we have to be here to feel this?' Those were his words when I read to him the line, 'I will make sure that he knows that his final resting place will be the place of his dreams.'

He then repeated a few times, 'You'll find it, Des, a glorious patch of green.' He often repeats things for dramatic effect, but I am impressed with the strength of emotion he feels for Ballycotton. He is desperate to be connected to Cork and to Ireland at the end.

I then pulled out Google maps and showed him Ballycotton on the satellite map. He was delighted to be looking at it again. It is so beautiful and I was impressed with my dad's taste. He has decided that he wants us to go to the lighthouse and, depending which way the wind is blowing, to just let his ashes drift out to the ocean on the breeze. He also wants us to sing 'The Old House', which is an old Irish song. I think it's a good choice, as it talks of a man coming back to where he is from and seeing everything abandoned. The final two lines have a strong resonance for me.

Why stand I here, like a ghost or a shadow?
It is time I was movin'; it is time I passed on.

Journal, 18 January 2011, Flushing, Queens

My dad asked the oncologist today if he had jumped the gun by stopping the chemo. He has felt invincible all day and now he feels like he can go on forever. My mother heard him ask the question. It is slightly unnerving to hear that he asked, because he never directly expresses to us that he is doubtful about his decision. But now I know for sure that he is.

We had a chat as a result and I told him what I thought. I think that he feels better as a result of being off chemo for a while now. The fact that he feels better is a victory. I feel it's a vindication of the decision because he is going to be able to enjoy some of the time he has left, rather than feeling sick all the time.

He seems happy with the decision, but I guess it's hard for anyone to accept that they are just allowing themselves to die. He actually said he feels guilty about just 'giving up'. I can't remember exactly what he said, but I got the impression he felt like he should be putting up a better fight for us. He also said he felt guilty that he was going to be a burden on us. In a way, it was a lovely thing that he would be worried about that. I guess he felt that by giving in it was in some way a lazy admission that he was now completely reliant on the help of his family and others.

It is tough to sort of argue in favour of death. You are not really doing that, but sometimes you hear the words coming out of your mouth and you fear that people might think you are rooting for your dad to die. I know I am arguing in favour of my father having less suffering and more quality of life, but when he seems to want to fight a little bit more, it can make you doubt yourself.

The most important thing though is being able to make sure my dad knows that he is not a burden at all. I just want to let him know that we love looking after him. It's even better to hear my mother say it. It was particularly nice today because she was so loving when she said it. It was not so much my mother saying, 'I will make sure everything gets done.' It was more like her saying, 'I will be with you, Mike, until the end.' I sometimes forget that underneath it all my mother loves my father very deeply.

Here they are, over forty years later, still together nearly every minute of the day. Here we all are, coming back together in the house we were raised in. That togetherness and that love were not always so evident. I can be so critical of what has been before, and I would not take back that criticism, but the challenges we faced as a family and the honesty with which we faced them have brought us to this point where we fight on together. It is just those tiny glimpses of love from my mother that I find so inspiring.

She must have called him Mike at that time. My mother mostly calls him Dad. Of course he is not her dad, he is our dad. When she calls him that I always think that she only sees him as the father of her children, as if she only sees him through the eyes of the family and not through the eyes of his lover.

Before we were born, she must have called him Mike. She must have because I know the energy was different then. My father said today, 'Your mother is very beautiful, isn't she?' What stood out was that she did not make a joke. It would have been like her to say, 'How many painkillers did you take today?' But she didn't, she didn't tap out.

I know that the moment stayed with them because it immediately inspired a nostalgic chat between my father and my mother about their life together before we were born. It was such a happy chat and I could see how happy they were together then. And I could see how happy my mother was to have been complimented in such a genuine way by my dad. I could see she felt beautiful when he said it. She felt loved. They loved each other. They love each other. You only get the odd glimpse of your parents' love for each other, but what a beautiful thing to see.

Journal, Saturday, 22 January 2011, 8.15 p.m. Backstage in Sligo during the Irish tour of My Dad Was Nearly James Bond. *Aidan is on stage*

The changes are coming faster than I expected. So much so that I am sitting backstage at a gig in Sligo just using this writing to make myself feel better about the awful news I heard today. I rang my mother, delighted with myself because I had spoken to my friend Mary, who is an oncologist and who has been advising us all along. She gave me a load of great advice about the best way to use hospice care and about asking the right questions about palliation.

It turns out they were answers to yesterday's questions because last night was the first night my dad was in real pain. He had unbearable pain in his thigh, which he had not experienced before last night. It could not have been any more real. Real pain showed real progression of the disease.

My mother was in a panic on the phone. No amount of painkillers alleviated the pain. She called the emergency number and they came with liquid morphine. According to my mother, he got no real relief from it. She sounded so scared and worried. I hate repeating myself, but when you are far away it is such a powerless feeling.

He screamed all night. My mother told me he asked if there was a way he could just have the plug pulled. Unfortunately he is not on life support, so that won't be happening. It's a terrible thing, cancer, and the way it takes you out.

I left New York two days ago, delighted with how he was feeling. Two days ago he was worried about giving up chemotherapy too early, and now he is screaming to die. I could not have imagined until this moment how unpredictable all this would be. I could not have imagined how horrible it would be. Perhaps he has been hiding certain amounts of pain from us recently, but this came on so heavy.

The poor guy. He is such a nice person and never harmed anyone in his entire lifetime. It seems so cruel that he should have to fight through all this pain at the end. We are made very badly, us humans. Why can't we just go when there is no point in living? I feel defeated, and the fight has only just begun.

I did not want to feel sorry for my dad. I don't know why I did not see that in the script. I just wanted to feel sad that I was going to lose him. I was enjoying appreciating what a great guy he was. The urgency had brought strange gifts. This is theft. This is ridiculous.

Journal, Wednesday, 26 January 2011, 12.35 p.m., Cork City

There are two main things that I want to write about. The first thing happened on Sunday, but I deliberately waited until now to write about it because it was such a powerful conversation with my dad that I did not want to try to make sense of it straight away but rather just let it be what it was. It is harder to remember now exactly what was said, but I could never have imagined that I would end up having a conversation like it with him.

The days before Sunday were horrible for my dad. After the pain, he was defeated. All he thinks about now is dying. He told me that if the pain continued, he would ask them to pull the plug. I think he kind of knew that it was not possible but, just in case, I reminded him that it was illegal. I did wonder, though, why a man who had lived a good life and had nothing left to live for but pain and reliance on others could not make the final call. I can understand if there is a chance of many more years, but all he wants to do is leave work a little early. He is not looking for a day off.

When I talked to him on Sunday he was finally comfortable and had been checked. His vital signs were all good and, to his disappointment, he was not on the way out the following day. The nurse had made clear to him that the pain he was feeling was from the cancer in his bones and that would not be the thing to kill him quickly. By the time I was talking to him he had been spending a lot of time thinking about dying.

I am not sure what the initial subject was, but I know that it came around to him telling me he had bad thoughts running around in his head. I was not sure what he meant, so I asked him to try to explain in some way. He told me that he was worried about the things he did in his life. I asked him if there was anything he felt guilty about. He said yes but did not offer any information. I was cool with not knowing whether I was the guy he wanted to tell or not. He had mentioned to me when I was home that a priest called Father Jim, who was also a member of AA, was due to call around to hear his confession, so I told him that if he was burdened by things he should tell Father Jim.

I asked him what kind of stuff he was worried about.

He mentioned things he had done when he was drinking. Knowing the programme of AA, I thought he had shared all of that stuff and had let it go. The more we talked, though, the more it became clear that it was less about what he had done and more about a deep belief that he was not a good person.

I can't remember the way he articulated all these thoughts. I just know that he told me that somewhere in him he felt like a bad person. He said he could not really put his finger on the feeling, but it was there. There was so much about this conversation that was familiar to me. I had had the same chats with counsellors and therapists over the years. I felt like I was listening to myself. I was definitely my father's son. So I said to him what was said to me, that it was shame he was feeling. I told him that it was a belief system he had programmed in him that he never escaped from.

He asked me why. I really did not want to be his therapist, I just wanted him to have relief. I can't remember the exact order of the things that were said, but I know I originally said that where it came from was not that important at this stage. What mattered was that he had the right to admit to himself that he was a good person. I then told him that, considering what he had achieved after the abuse he had received as a child and the love that he had shown his family, he was, in fact, a great person. I think I told him that he was one of the greatest people that ever lived.

He said that it was a good point. He said that it would be possible to look at it that way. So I said it didn't matter what his mother had done to him or anything else that was eating away at him; all he had to do was give himself a break and admit that he was a good person. I then told him that he could even say it right now on the phone. He said that he could not do that. He then said something to the effect of him not deserving it or believing it.

I am not sure if I got angry, but I know I got passionate. I said that it was up to him. He had the power to liberate himself because it was only what *he* felt now that mattered. I pleaded with him to give himself a break just this once and allow himself to say he was a good person. I told him that everyone he knew worshipped him. I told him that my whole life everyone always told me how amazing my dad was. People always raved about how our dad was the nicest man. Everyone he was ever involved with thought he was a great man, except for him. So I pleaded that now, at the end, the most important thing was that he left this world with the certainty that he knew he was a good man. As part of the evidence to back up my case, somewhere in the conversation I told him that I could not love him more.

I was not just trying to get him to say this as a surface exercise. I could feel him on the cliff edge of a major admission. I knew that this was part of who he was. I knew that he carried this negative view of himself around, and I knew it motivated much of his behaviour. I recognized that I had been at similar points when I'd fought to say a simple sentence because I knew it had power in the moment. I wanted him to begin the process of freedom from that prison.

I am not good enough! Such a simple sentence. How could so much of what hurts us be that simple?

He told me he was a good person.

'Damn fucking right you are!' I said.

I admitted to him after that that I pretty much just copied what a therapist had done with me around the same beliefs. I would not belittle what I have been through in my life. In fact, it's no surprise I ended up with the same doubts about my worth on the planet as my father. But whatever I had to deal with in a therapist's office is nothing compared to the trauma that my dad experienced. I told him that he had to remind himself every day from here on in that he was a great person and that he was good enough. I told him he was not allowed to leave this life with any doubts about that.

I felt so lucky in a way to have a dad who could talk so openly about things. It made his imminent death seem like such an opportunity for us. We cannot be any closer now.

40

The week of shows in Cork as my father lay dying was very powerful. Essentially I was performing every night, hoping he was not going to go too fast. One thing I wanted to do while I was in Cork was to go down to Ballycotton to film footage of places my dad might like as his final resting place. He had told me many times, and he said it in an interview on the documentary, that he wanted his ashes spread in Ballycotton.

He said, 'There is a field next to the cliffs up there in Ballycotton, you could see right out on to the lighthouse. I used to go mushrooming there when I was a lad. I am sure there are all houses there now.' As I mentioned, we had discussed the spot in greater detail in more recent times, but I wanted to have something to show him when I got back to New York. I had always thought my dad's memory would not be right about where he was thinking, but after the documentary was shown I got tons of emails talking about the exact spot he was talking about. Every one said the same place.

Pat Kiernan, a theatre director from Cork whom I very much admire, had come to see the show one of the nights after the documentary had been broadcast. Once again he knew exactly where I was talking about, and he had his own story about a time when he had been exploring the cliff walk in Ballycotton himself. He told me there was a set of steps down the cliff towards the sea, about half a mile from the town. If I took the steps all the way down I would find a little swimming hole. He said when he had found it he thought it was quite an amazing place, and when he met one of the locals they told him that traditionally it was known as 'the paradise'. He was adamant that I go there. Before even seeing it I was convinced that this was the spot in my dad's head. I also thought that there was something intense about the conversation with Pat; I felt that maybe we were meant to have this conversation. I also felt right that the show should finish in Cork, close to where my father always thought was paradise.

So I went to the paradise with my best friend, Ian. We walked along the cliff walk, and it was just as my dad had described it, with the lighthouse in the distance. There is something remarkable about the cliff walk because all you can see is the vast ocean and the cliffs beyond heading west. It is not like most of the East Cork coastline, which is tamer. It has a strength and power that is more like West Cork.

As we walked down the steps, I could hear the ocean hammering against the rocks. It felt wild and rocky and dangerous. But when I got to the bottom it had a tiny protected pool of deep water, and just beyond a few rocks was the ocean spraying high and white, showering the pool. This was indeed a paradise; there is nothing I like more than to be as close as possible to the untamed sea. It humbles me.

It was a perfect place. I filmed the spot, saying a few words to my dad about how we might set him off on his final journey. I told him I would dive in after him and have one final swim in the ocean together, as we had done in Westhampton and at the Forty Foot in Sandycove, Dublin, a few Christmases before. I liked the thought of one final swim together in Cork. One final swim together in Ireland, a place to which we both escaped and where we both found peace. I liked the paradise because it was not protected enough to be stagnant in any way. You could see the water being sucked out and thrust back in with the ebb and flow of the tide. I knew that I could step back out and continue the journey and he would not be stuck there in the pool; he would get sucked straight out into the vast expanse of the sea.

(I have yet to go down those steps with my brothers and my mother. We have not found the right time yet. I don't even think I want to yet. It's nice to think that there is one more thing to look forward to when the show is over. There is still one final day to say goodbye.)

41

Journal, Friday, 28 January 2011, 1.30 a.m. Back in the hotel in Cork City

Just got off the phone after my mother rang me today and I could tell she was upset. She began the conversation by saying in a strained tone, 'Not a good day today.' I asked her what had happened, assuming it was more problems with constipation or nausea or pain. There was silence on the phone. The pause lasted for quite a few seconds. She did not have to say anything after that; the pause spoke volumes. I knew it was the calm before the storm. I knew the rest of what my mother would say would come with tears.

'The hospice nurse came today and she says that seeing how much he has declined since last week, that he only has two to four weeks, maybe even less.' She completely broke down then and just handed the phone to the nurse. My mother hates having to talk about the bad news. I felt worse for my mother than I did for my dad. Sympathy aside though, I would have preferred not to talk to the nurse right then and there without warning as I was a tad emotional, but I had no choice as seconds later she was on the phone.

It's hard to talk on the phone to someone you don't know about how long your father has to live. She introduced herself as the hospice nurse and then said, 'Do you have any questions?' I actually did not have any questions because I was in shock. So I just told her what I was actually feeling. I said, 'Actually, my mother just told me you said my dad only has a short time and handed the phone to you as she was crying.'

She told me that my mother was concerned that I would not have enough time to get back, seeing as I was abroad. She then gave me the details of why she thought his time was short. I felt compelled to tell her that this was tough for my mother, as she has never truly accepted that this day was coming and that was probably why she handed her the phone in such haste. I don't know why I told her this, but I guess I was just trying to let her know why I was unprepared for the conversation. That is definitely a bit of my dad in me, that I was concerned about what this woman would think about the little drama that preceded her talking to me.

She told me that my dad would be getting methadone which, though more closely associated with heroin maintenance, was a very good pain reliever in this situation. I asked her when he would be going on the morphine drip, and she told me that would not happen as he was staying at home. She was nice and informative, and that was it. I asked to be put back on to my mother.

I should have asked my mother to take a picture of that woman. When I got off the phone I wondered where she was from. I did not know if she was white or black or Asian. It does not really matter, but it seems like a weird thing to talk to someone on the phone about such important information and not have a clue who they are. It's fine when you are complaining about your phone bill, but it just seems a bit cold when you are talking about how long your father has to live. It's a perfect example of how being far away is a horrible thing as the time gets closer.

My mother got back on the phone and she was still crying. I think she did one of her very open diaphragm 'Oh God, Des!' exclamations. It's such a distinct way that my mother has of doing it. Sometimes it's followed by, 'What are we going to do?' but I don't think she said that. Then she asked me, 'Are you OK?' and honestly I was OK at that moment. I told her that it was good news because all Dad talked about now was wanting to die. She then said that if I was OK then she would be fine. She had been so worried about me being far away and hearing the news. I could hear the relief in her voice.

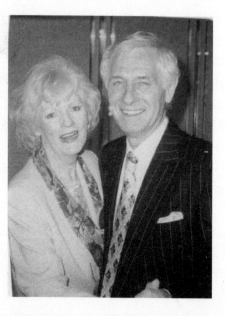

She told me she just wanted three weeks. She felt she needed that time to get her head around it. I told her that I would be fine if he died tomorrow because that's what he wants. I tried to reassure her that if he died tomorrow and I was in Ireland, that I would be content because I had said everything I wanted to say and that I could not love the man any more than I did right at that moment. Coincidentally, I could not have loved my mother more than at that moment either. Maybe it's silly, because I know my mother worries about me all the time, but not in the way she was worried about me then. She wasn't worried about me being in trouble or being stressed; she was worried about how I felt. She was being very loving, and I could feel it. I was really loving her too, and not out of obligation.

Journal, Saturday evening, 29 January 2011

Later this evening I was backstage at the Cork Opera House for about twenty minutes before the opening act (who was standing in for Aidan) was due to go on. I told my mother my plan to come home for a few days to make sure that I could see my dad before he lost consciousness, and then I'd decide what to do. She was delighted that I was coming home, but hated me having to cancel shows. My mother's fear of death is only outweighed by her fear that my career will implode any day.

We chatted for a while, but only one thing really mattered. She told me that she did not see how he had such a short time because his breathing was so good. She had been up all last night, listening to his breathing. For ages she just listened to it. Then he started snoring and she told me that for most of their lives together she hated him snoring, but she thought last night that it was the loveliest sound and she wished she could hear it forever. It was a sad but lovely thought. Just her desire to be with him was so lovely. I am going to miss him too, no doubt, but I will always remember how I realized how much my parents loved each other by hearing their openness in these last few weeks.

I am lucky really because we are genuinely open at the moment. I know perhaps this is not the norm, but I am loving it. My mother told me that my father always denied he snored and she never woke him up, no matter how bad the noise, yet any time she snored he would wake her up straight away. 'Eileen, you are snoring!' I laughed, particularly at the way she told the story. I laughed also because she does not realize that she snores every night.

Journal, Wednesday, 2 February 2011, 4 a.m. Flushing, Queens, New York

I made it back after some serious drama trying to get here. My flight had been cancelled as JFK was closed. I was in a major panic because Aidan had told me the night before that my father was close to death and that I should try to get escorted through immigration if I could, just in case it was coming down to hours. I actually got mad at him because you do immigration in Dublin so it would not have made a difference and it just panicked me beyond belief. So when the flight got cancelled I was freaking out. In the end I just got a flight to Philadelphia and drove to New York. It was pretty exciting in the end, running around the airport. I will always remember that Metallica's 'Nothing Else Matters' was in my head the whole time I was running around because I had decided that nothing else mattered other than getting home.

I made it and I was finally back with my dad. I walked into the room and I could see how far he had declined in the last two and a half weeks. He opened his eyes and the first thing he said was, 'Des.' He knew me straight away and that was all that mattered. I was glad he knew I was there. I knew he had lost the ability to communicate properly, but he was so quick in seeing me that I knew it had registered that his whole family were home to be with him.

Of course I cried. It is sad to see someone so close to death. Death is all over him now. His hands and arms are in the air and his eyes have a glassed-over look. He speaks to people who are not there and he always uses an Irish accent when he speaks. I think it will only be a day or two, to be honest. Today I don't find the emotion overwhelming because I am just so glad to be home. After days of feeling so far away and having to hear news over the phone about him getting worse, the fact that I am downstairs and can actually hear his heavy breaths while I write this feels like paradise.

There is nothing left to do. There is nothing I wish we could have done. It's all about making sure he can fly.

Journal, Thursday, 3 February 2011, Flushing, Queens

He is hanging around now, stuck in this near-death state. Every now and then you get a little glimpse of his old self. It usually comes when someone visits. It's as if he is saving all his energy so that he has a little bit to give when someone comes over. At the very end the most important thing is the performance and making sure that other people are comfortable.

I feel strange saying it, but there is something quite fun about all this. It's great to see all the people and talk to my dad's old friends on the phone. We are in the presence of relentless and powerful praise of my father, coming at us from all angles. It seems very genuine and the circumstances bring out very strong emotions in people. I feel charged up with something very fundamental. All the things that matter are present: love, family, compassion, companionship and loyalty. When you feel them so strongly together it's easy to feel, despite the sadness, that this is really a celebration. That we are witnessing the end of a great performance with each phone call and visit like a standing ovation or shout for an encore. People really loved my dad.

My cousin Dennis, who is the son of my mother's sister Carol, said the most amazing thing yesterday. He said that he never saw my dad as an uncle through marriage. To him my dad was always his uncle of blood. The connection people had with him becomes so clear when you hear people speak like that.

I have also enjoyed having to call his friends. I think that is because when you put the phone to my dad's ear and tell him who it is, he really perks up. People from his long-gone past perk him up the most, as I think that is where he spends most of his time at the moment. For two months I have been trying to get a hold of Dudley Sutton, his buddy from London. My dad really wanted to talk to him. I would have preferred to get a hold of him when my dad could really talk, but in the end it probably worked out because it was so uplifting to catch a glimpse of the old dad when I put the phone to his ear.

His accent went real London real quick. 'Dudley, hello, mate. Hello, my son.' Dudley said a few things in his ear and there was not much after that but I told him to say goodbye to Dudley and he said, ''Bye, Dudley, 'bye, my son.' It was great because it proved that he could still hear us. It proved that in some way he still knew what was going on.

But it also proved something else: that even in the end he would always be the person he was talking to. We joked about that all our lives. Depending on who was on the phone would determine my dad's accent. I do it myself to a certain extent and I realize that sometimes you don't even mean to do it. But I was surprised that it was still happening on his deathbed. Tony Kearns from Midleton rang today, and straight away he was a Cork man. Everything finished with 'boy'. 'All right, boy! Sound out!' No more 'my son' or 'mate'. When I heard on the phone how Tony Kearns talked about my dad, I realized that these men really had been best friends. They were little divils running around Midleton together. I know that it is Ireland he is going back to in his head. It really is who he is.

Journal, Saturday, 5 February 2011

My dad died yesterday morning. I was there with him, along with my family. In the end, amidst the refrain of the 'death rattle', we all slept in the room. My mother was in the bed adjacent to my father, and my two brothers and I slept wrapped in duvets on the floor. It was such a sad but wonderful thing that we would end up together like three scared boys looking for the safety of our parents' room to get us through the night. I was not scared, though. I was there to make sure my dad was not scared to go. I rubbed his head for two days and told him he was free to go. We all told him we would look after Mom and that he had lived a great life. I told him he would be leaving this world surrounded in love.

Most importantly, I repeated over and over that he was a good person. I know he left this world sure of that.

It's tough to listen to the final grasp on life. You just wish you could clear his throat for him and then it happens. You can look up the process online if you like. My dad followed the stages by the book. But you can't look up what that moment is like for you.

The power of the victory.

The end of a life well lived.

There is a sense of being as close as you can be to the essence of humanity. In the end there is death and the legacy of your life. But when you take that last breath with the awe and wonder of your children praising you intensely right in your eyes, it must be the ultimate end to your humanity. These are the things that really matter.

You did it, man. That's what we shouted at him. You did it. We actually thought he was gone already when twenty seconds later he had one last gasp. We were already crying, so we got a fright and then we laughed for about thirty seconds. It was the funniest thing. I then rubbed his head and felt the sweat and the warmth still there. He is not gone straight away. It is too immediate for you to feel that way. So we enjoyed that time. We cried and we joked and we even had some jokes with him. Why would we not take the piss out of him in the end? We had done so all our lives.

I washed him up a little bit and tried to get his face sitting a bit straighter, in case people came by. He would have wanted it that way. We then waited for the logistics of death to help us say goodbye.

42

After my dad died we had asked Tom Brick to organize everything for us. Tom is a local man from St Kevin's who is in the funeral game. He also lost his son, a fireman who died in a factory fire in the Bronx. It was a big story in our area because he was the first fireman to die after 9/11. I felt comforted, knowing that someone who had dealt with death on such a tragic level was helping us to deal with our loss.

While we were waiting for the funeral home guys to load up my dad in the van, Mr Brick said to me that nobody does death better than the Irish. Now you have to remember that in America we are Irish. There is no Irish-American label thrown around in everyday conversation. I feel he is right, though. I think death shows off Irish people's ability to deal with tragedy and crisis. It definitely shows off their ability to be funny about it.

My dad had that sense of humour about death always. A few months before he died he asked me if I would continue to do the show after he died. I really did not know if I would be able to as I was clueless about how grief would affect me. I should have known that he was not too worried about me being able to do the show or not; this was just his way of letting me know that he had a funny idea about what I could do at the end of the show after he had died.

He suggested that I film in a graveyard. He had a very detailed picture in his mind. He said: 'I want you to do a wide shot over the entire graveyard to establish where you are. Then I want you to pan down and zoom in on my gravestone. Now there won't be one because I am being cremated, so you will have to make one up. On the gravestone it should say,

MIKE BISHOP

1936–201X

HE STORMED IT

'I want you to hold that shot for about five or six seconds and then I want you to pan down and Black Bob will be lying on top of the grave, missing his master.'

I thought that was flipping hilarious. I loved it because he had totally grasped the concept of the call-back in comedy. It's such a simple trick, but to use it about your own death is bloody genius. I may have said this before but it's worth repeating: my dad impressed me so much throughout the whole process. I had thought of him as a fool for most of my life, but, boy, when he stepped up was he a warrior.

His other great moment of funeral humour came after the bitter-sweet occasion of Kathleen Kearney dying. Kathleen was the wife of my dad's best friend, Jim. Even writing his name down now makes me sad, because so much of my grief is triggered by how close I realized those two men were at the end of my dad's life. Their friendship was such a wonderful thing. Jim actually got up at my dad's wake and said the most beautifully simple thing. 'Mike was the best friend I ever had.' When you hear that coming from a strong man like Jim Kearney, who once played hurling for County Clare in the 1950s, you know it comes from the heart. He sat for a few hours a day at the end, just looking at my dad and wanting to be near him. I suppose he was watching a lot of people disappear around him.

Anyway, Jim's wife died and it was a sad and joyful day

because she had suffered with Alzheimer's for many years. They had really said goodbye to her years earlier, but it was a sad occasion. It was a big song-and-dance getting my dad ready, because he was insistent on dressing up properly for it. I told him people would understand if he just wore his black sweat-pants and a sweater, but he was having none of it. He was so puffed up from all the drugs and his feet were swollen, so it took us ages to get him ready. There was not a hope that he was going to get his trousers shut, so he had to leave them open and close his pants with a belt. Eventually he was ready, and once he got his breath back he said, 'This is like a dress rehearsal!'

My mother hated that joke because she still did not like to contemplate the inevitable, but I thought it was brilliant.

I think my favourite joke in the circumstances came from Aidan on the morning of my dad's funeral. We were at the funeral home, getting ready to say goodbye to my dad for the last time before they closed the casket before the funeral Mass. It is one of the tougher moments and I remembered from my nan's funeral that when you have to say goodbye everybody breaks down. You also have to be told about the logistics of what is going to happen and asked if there is anything you want to put in the coffin. My Aunt Mary insisted, with my mother's support, that my dad have rosary beads. We put in flowers from my nephew Kieran and we draped him in his Cork hurling jersey that he had requested be near him when he was laid out.

During this discussion I asked Mr Brick if they took off my dad's suit before the cremation. He said that we should take off his ring and anything else we wanted to keep before we left, that everything else would go for incineration with him. So Aidan said, 'They burn everything. Damn, if I'd known that I would have brought a few bags of garbage to throw in there.' It was funny anyway, but it was doubly funny because my dad in New York and Aidan in Dublin both obsessed about garbage day. They were father and son on that front: a fitting joke for them to share together in the end.

Mr Brick told us that an entire new chapter in his professional life had been written as a result of his experience dealing with us through the whole process – such a nice thing to say. He was really amazing. The pall that draped my dad's coffin in the church had actually been donated by Mr Brick to the church and had been the pall that draped his son Tom's coffin. Tom's name is on it. There was so much community strength in all that. Another dad impressed me that day.

43

My dad's death was very public in the end. He died eight days after the documentary came out, so the Irish press charted the days from when I had to cancel shows to come home, to the news that he had passed away. We did not mind that because, being the man he was, we knew that he would have been delighted with the press attention. It would have been especially satisfying for my dad if he had seen the article in the *Examiner* with the headline, 'Cork Comedian's Father Dies'. The *Examiner* might not have realized how much that meant to me either.

My mother was adamant that I get back to performing the show as soon as possible. I am not sure why she thought that was the right thing to do, but she was of the firm belief that everyone should try to get back to their normal routine. That is good advice, but it's tough when your normal routine is doing a stand-up show about your dying father who has now just died. I flew back to Ireland still very much on the strange buzz you feel after the funeral. From the moment I got on the plane I was dealing with the strange phenomenon of everyone knowing that my dad had died because it had been all over the news. 'Really sorry to hear about your dad.' 'My condolences.' It is kind of like being stuck in the funeral for an extended period because you have to thank a load of people you don't know over and over and over.

I had only one night at home in Dublin, and suddenly I was in Galway, getting ready to do the show, not even a week after my dad had died. The adrenalin of the funeral was still pumping through me. I did not think much about things until the moment when I was standing backstage. The James Bond ski film-clips that I always show as the crowd was coming in were playing. 'Goldfinger' was blaring over the clips and then we got clearance. As soon as I heard the hum of Zulu warriors rising from the opening clip of the show, which is my dad's small scene from *Zulu*, it hit me. This young man on the screen is my dad and he is now dead. The enormity of life and death smacked me in the face. The nerves of performing and the grief were pulsating through me. As the clip played I had only one thought: 'All this time I have been preparing for death and now that it is here I am unprepared.' I really wasn't preparing for death, I was trying to make the most of life.

I had no time to dwell on it. My next thought was, 'This is going to be really tough.' I announced myself and walked out on to the stage. The applause was deafening. I had done the show many times, but this was a special welcome. I could feel it strongly and it was not helping. I bowed and stayed down for an extra few seconds. The show must go on, Dad!

44

Years ago, when I first started talking to my dad about the original version of *My Dad Was Nearly James Bond*, I was drilling him pretty hard about how true the whole story was. I still had a lot of doubts about my dad's stories and I couldn't bring all this to the public and then find out he had been making it up all along. He reminded me of the celebrated article that someone was supposed to have in Midleton about how he was in the running for the Bond role. The heading of the mythical piece was something like, 'The Irish Man Who Was Nearly James Bond' (to be honest, it was most likely my inspiration for the show title). I must have heard people describing this story for years in Midleton. It was part of the legend that had grown up around my dad. But no one ever produced it. My dad said it had been written by an Irish actor and journalist, Vass Anderson. Vass had been in the production of *Sive* that the Bond people had allegedly attended to see my father.

When I decided to do the show in the UK I tried to get more background from my dad about Vass Anderson, particularly after he got sick, so I needed to be sure this story was not complete bullshit. I looked him up on the internet and saw his name mentioned in passing in an article or two about Irish writers. He had parts in plenty of movies and TV shows, but I could not get a contact. I put it out on Twitter and on Facebook, but nobody got back to me about him. Nobody in Midleton could even remember who had the original article or where it had appeared. At some stage I gave up trying to find Vass Anderson and the article. It was not integral to the story, but it just would have been great to see it in print.

In May 2011 I brought the show to the Soho Theatre in London for two weeks. It felt wonderful to bring it back to London, and in particular to the West End. My father's journey with me began in London and it was nice to take our journey together back there for a little encore. I was sad he had not been able to come back with me, but in a way that is what we were doing with the show. The run went great.

One night I arrived back in the dressing room to find a letter that had been posted to me at the venue. The letter had a London address at the top and it was typed on an old-fashioned typewriter. It was from Vass Anderson.

He said he was delighted to read the review of the show in the *Evening Standard* but very sad to hear of my dad's passing. He said he knew my dad well and did a show with him in a theatre on St Martin's Lane when my dad was trying to get acting experience. He said that he wrote an article about him for the *Irish Post* as a result of him being part-Irish and how he was nearly James Bond. He said he remembered my dad as a very gentle man and described going to the opening of his then wife's shop in Chelsea.

I did not pay much attention to the wife bit. I knew that for a time my father had a serious girlfriend called Valerie, that she had been back to Midleton with him a few times and that they had a hairdressing salon together in Chelsea. He was annoyed that the business wasn't a success, but I always got the impression that there was something not quite right with that part of his entrepreneurial history. His recollections definitely came across as being sourced from the regret part of his brain.

I thought it was great that I had finally found Vass and

that the story of the newspaper article was true. I was sad, though, that he had to find out about my father the way he did. I was sad too because of how he described my father: 'a gentle man'. That really touched me. That was quite a specific thing to remember about him, and it was definitely true. The fact that the letter was typed on an old typewriter only added to the quaintness of it and it was an incredible letter to get.

I told my mother about it and she kind of remembered his name. She could not remember if it was from the newspaper piece or from actually meeting him.

What I did not anticipate was her shock at him mentioning Dad's wife. It turned out that my father had indeed been married before and he had told my mother he never wanted us to know. The marriage did not last very long, but Valerie had been his wife. My father was separated from her but still married when he met my mother. When he decided he wanted to marry my mother, he had to get Valerie to agree to the divorce, but she would not agree unless he signed over his half of the shop to her. I got the impression from my mother that this really pissed him off because I assume it was money from his modelling success that had funded it from the beginning. But he signed it over to her so he could move on with his life and marry my mother.

My mother knew about all this and had met Valerie. They should have never got married in the first place. There was a lot of booze involved in their relationship, and Valerie died of alcoholism in the 1990s. Her sister had called our house to let my dad know when she died. Her parents were Irish and my father had gotten along very well with them.

We had no idea about this. Not even at the end, when I thought my dad had got everything off his chest, did he tell us about this. I would like to think that this was not really on his mind, but he repeated to my mother in those final weeks what they had agreed throughout their whole life, that even after he died he did not want his boys to know that he had once been married and had got a divorce. I don't know why he did not want us to know. My dad was funny like that sometimes, and would worry about things that were really quite trivial.

I guess my mother decided to tell me after the letter and also because I had been trying to piece together parts of my dad's story that were hard to figure out based on the fragmented timelines and his desire to embellish everything. I don't think she felt bad about telling me. I thought it was funny that even in the end when my dad had called his musical *Secrets* he would still hold on to one more. And even though he wrote a song called 'Redeem Me', he still felt a little shame about something.

I have spoken to Vass since I received that letter and he has a razor-sharp memory for his age. He not only remembers Valerie well but recalls the night they had the official opening of the beauty salon. He told me it was a very exciting affair and many celebrities of the time were there. He told me Valerie was really into being part of the trendy London scene of that time, that she was quite a pushy woman and he was not surprised to find out that my dad lost out over the shop. 'I am not surprised, being who she was, that she ran business rings around him,' he said.

It all makes sense, because I think my dad was quite sore all his life about getting screwed out of that business. It explains why he would get irrationally annoyed when talking about what could have been. I don't know all the details, but I assume he must have put quite a lot of what he had made up until that point into the shop, and it all disappeared. That is quite an understandable thing to find difficult to get over.

My mother also told me that she was pretty sure that

Valerie ended up having an affair with the manager of the salon and that is why they broke up before he went to New York. It may be one of the motivations for why he left. I found out all of this after he died, so I will never know.

Trying to piece together my dad's story has been sort of like trying to figure out a password. Trying to do it justice has been like doing sudoku. When you think you finally have a handle on what is real and what is a rewrite, you find out another massive piece of drama. For instance, another thing we discovered in the last few months of my dad's life was that his father Stanley was born out of wedlock and never knew his father. I mention this because my father lived his whole life believing his grandfather died in the Battle of the Somme. He also grew up believing that Bishop was his grandfather's name, whereas it was actually his grandmother's name. It is amazing how such massive bits of information that are so intimately connected to you can be kept from you for so long. Not that it was a terrible deception, but it was a final injustice in a traumatic family story. These are big revelations. This story is epic. Some might not even believe all this happened to one man. The joke of it all is, I used to make fun of him for trying to write the great epic musical spanning three generations. I used to call him Leon Uris with a banjo. I can't see why he did not look to his own life, because what is more epic than the many lives he had and the dramas he survived?

45

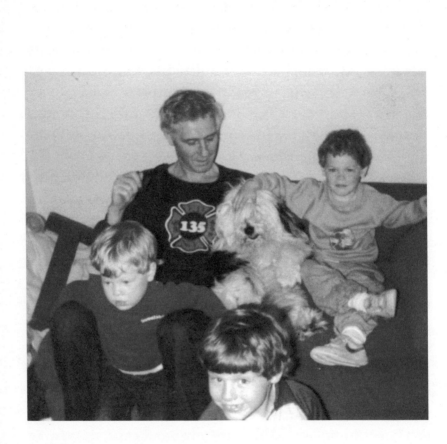

Journal, 29 May 2011. Flushing, Queens

Coming home for the first time since my dad's funeral
has been hard. I rented a car for this trip because I was
going to head out to Westhampton to finish off this very
book I am writing right now. So I was on my own, driving
down Union Turnpike towards 188th Street. It was such a
familiar journey home from JFK airport. It was the sights
of coming home from Ireland I was looking at. Driving

in that direction on Union Turnpike always meant I was just about to see my brothers and my father again. It was always my mother driving.

I had to drive past the chemo place. I stared at it in the late May heat and I could see the piles of dirty snow on the kerb at the bus stop and me holding my dad's hand as he navigated through a gap and waddled to the doorway.

We had three dogs in our lives, but two of them had a very strong presence. The first was Scruffy (in the picture above) and he was the most loving dog ever. Our second dog was Mistress and she was wild, but she matured into the most dynamic animal. She barked a lot, though. Mistress used to bark like crazy when she realized I was home. She would jump all over me and then I would go and hug Scruffy, who was more like my brother than a dog.

Scruffy died after we put him to sleep in the Easter of 1992. He had gotten very old and we decided to do it as a family while I was back from school. We stayed in the room while the injection was administered and I will never forget the difference between his body only seconds before and his lifeless head. He was gone immediately and I found it very profound. It was my first real encounter with death.

Mistress lived on for years after that and did not die until a few years ago. I happened to be home then also, as she seemed to be dying before our eyes. The night before we had her put down she was in so much pain that every time she fell asleep she would jerk awake from the pain of her body lying down. I slid my body in between her legs so that when she fell asleep she would not drop and the pain in her hips would ease. That night she slept on me for ages, and I fell asleep myself. When she woke up she kept going into corners and I later read that was a sign she was ready to die.

She was so light, I carried her to the vet with my dad that morning. I could not wait anymore as I had spent much of the night pondering a way to end her misery myself, but I did not know how to do it. She was so calm as I held her and I could feel that she had given up. She was really only hair and bones. She weighed twenty-six pounds and was riddled with cancer.

The vet told us we were doing the right thing, and once again I stayed with her as she said goodbye. My brother Michael John was angry with me because I did not wait for him to be there, but he was working and both myself and my dad felt we had to do it there and then.

It was one of the saddest things to come home that first time from Ireland after that and not hear the barks. It was terrible not to be welcomed home by crazy Mistress and be covered in her white hair. It almost seemed strange that the first thing I had to do when I came home was not to wipe dog hair off my jeans. I still hear her bark every time I come home, despite all the years that have passed.

I thought of her bark when I got home a few days ago. I knew that for the first time I was not going to walk into the living room and see my dad get up from his chair and hug me. I knew I was not going to go up to the room, as had been my more recent habit, and see how he was doing. It was a grief I have never known before.

Before I walked into the house on my own I listened because it was that quiet time of the day. The Aer Lingus flight gets you in so that you get back to the house around two o'clock in the afternoon. There was no one around and it was quiet. The leaves were back on the trees and the late spring brightness had returned to what was barren and grey when I had left, a few months before. I could hear the leaves from the same trees that had soothed me my whole life and I could see the clothes hanging in the same empty alleyways.

Acknowledgements

There have many people involved in the journey of telling my dad's story. I would like to thank my editor Patricia Deevy, Michael McLoughlin and all in Penguin for making this happen, and Faith O'Grady for always asking me when I was going to write a book. Richard and all in Lisa Richards and all at Off the Kerb for the UK tour, Pat Comer for making an awesome documentary, Mick Burke for keeping the live show going, Cathal Murray for coming along for the ride, Conal Morrison for directing the live show. Big thanks to Aunt Mary, Uncle Jack and Aunt Peg for sharing their lives too, and my Aunt Joan in particular. Thanks to the fourteen other grandkids of Flushing. Always thanks to the Gibneys for being a home away from home. Pete Venetis for filming in church. Thanks to all at the Assembly Rooms for making my dad feel like a star, Flee, Eddie, Joss, Aoife, Kelan, Ruth and Liz for putting Edinburgh together. Thanks to the *Bexhill Observer*, Vass Anderson, Terry Maidment (Come on, the Blues!). Thanks to all my cousins in Midleton for all the stories. Ed Torres for the funeral especially, Jim Kearney for being my dad's best friend. Thanks to Bill and Bob for all the advice. Thanks to Jason Byrne, John Bishop, Maeve Higgins, Dave O'Doherty, Shappi Korsandi, Michael Mee, Adam Hilils and all the comedians who championed the live show and Steve Bennett for the advising review and Richard Bacon for his public praise. Also Bec And Aillie for helping me through the early shows in Oz. Thanks to Brian Quinn for the graphics. Mugsy for being Black Bob. Thanks to Kieran and Conor who will one day be old enough to think it's cool to be thanked. Thanks to Jenny Lee Masterson for being so chilled in the chaos. David Simon for the escape. Willy and PJ and all the neighbours who were so awesome with the food and the well-wishing. Thanks to all the Westhampton crew. Thanks to Tom Brick, and to the Sullivans I say football is being discussed in the sky. To Ian Dorgan and Pat Kiernan for the Paradise. Thanks to little Jenny for her card. Thanks to Mary Morrogh for being my personal cancer adviser and Nicky for texting me her number every time I lost it. Finally, to Dr Fulman and all at Queens medical for buying us some time. Sweet!